For the Centuries

St. Elizabeth Healthcare and
Northern Kentucky *1861–2011*

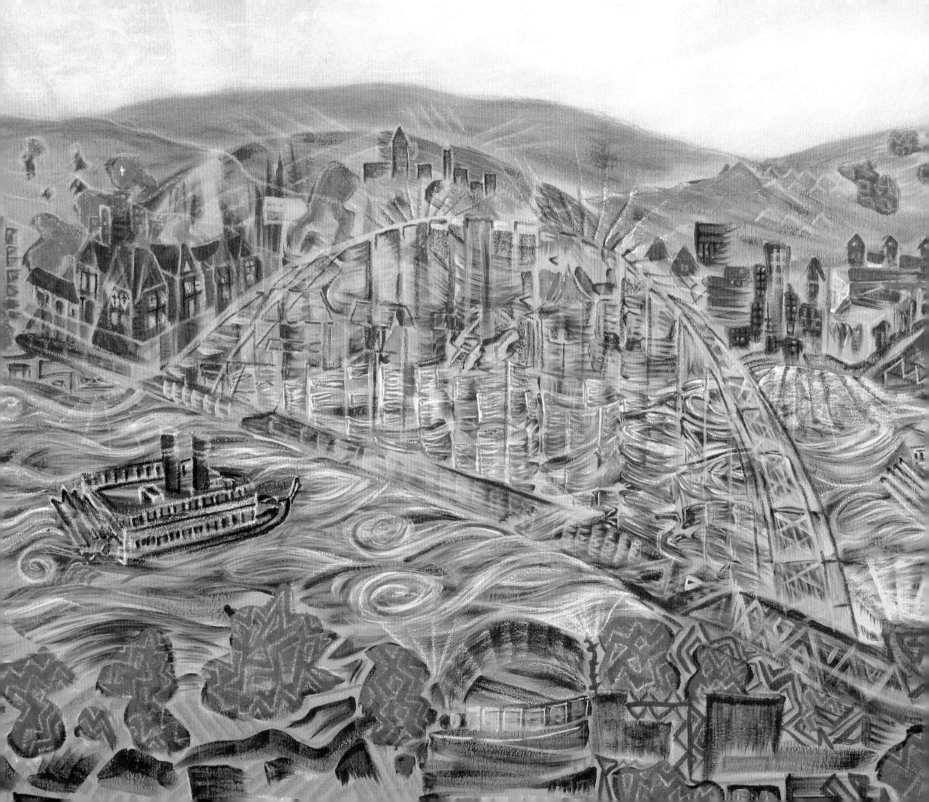

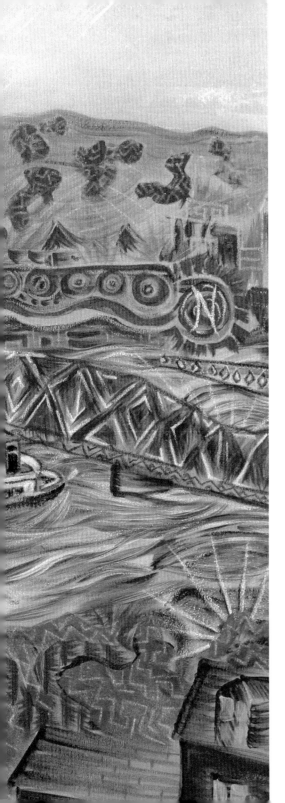

For the Centuries

St. Elizabeth Healthcare and
Northern Kentucky *1861-2011*

Brian L. Hackett, Ph. D.

With contributions by
Paul Tenkotte, Ph. D. and Rebecca Bailey, Ph. D.

For the Centuries: St. Elizabeth Healthcare and Northern Kentucky 1861–2011

Copyright © 2011 St. Elizabeth Healthcare
All rights reserved

First edition

No part of this book may be reproduced in any form or by an electronic
or mechanical means, including information storage and retrieval
systems, without permission in writing from St. Elizabeth Healthcare,
except by a reviewer who may quote brief passages in a review.

ISBN: 978-0-615-46670-5

Written by Brian L. Hackett, Ph. D. with Paul Tenkotte, Ph. D. and Rebecca Bailey, Ph. D.

Designed by Scott Bruno, b graphic design • *b-graphicdesign.com*

Printed and bound in the United States of America
by The C J Krehbiel Company, Cincinnati, OH 45227 • *cjkusa.com*

Cover art by Michael C. Burns IV of *MuralPop.com*

This book is dedicated to the St. Elizabeth Healthcare volunteers and family, of yesterday and today, for all of the lives they have saved, the hurt they have eased, and the community they have built. Thank you for being there for us for over 150 years.

ST. ELIZABETH HOSPITAL, 21st AND EASTERN AVENUE, COVINGTON, KY.—5

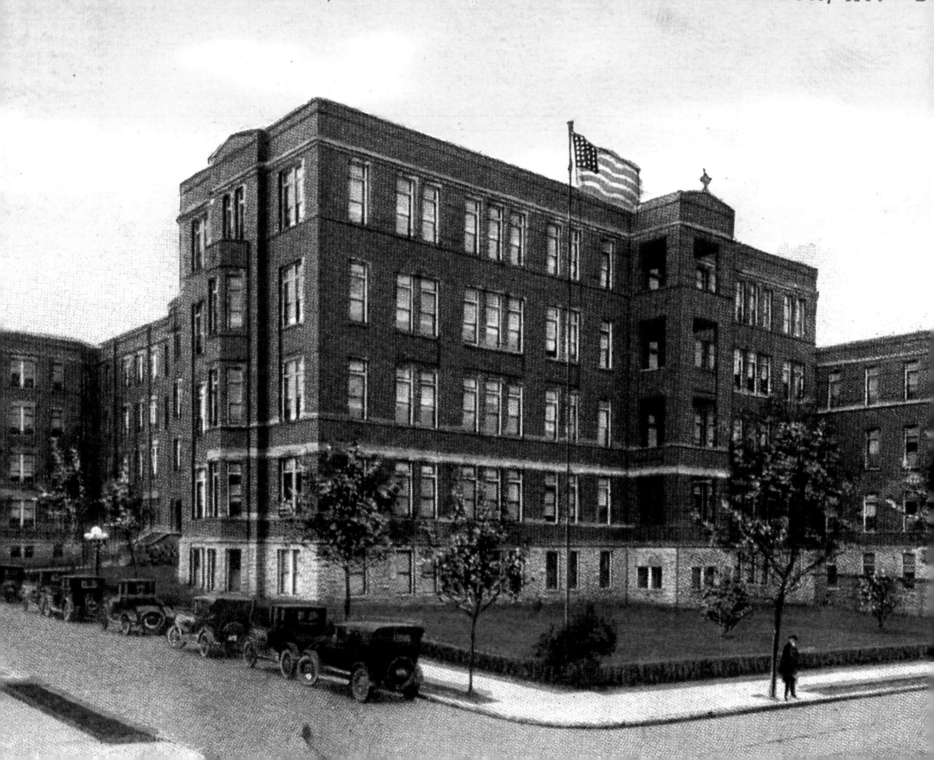

Contents

A special thanks to those individuals whose efforts made this book possible.

Veronica Buchanan	Michele Halloran
Donald Clare	Gary Hartwig
Denise Clarke	Ruth Henthorn
Travis Collins	Mary Milburn
Sister Mary	Anita Murphy
Jacinta Doyle, SFP	Emily Prabell
Cierra Earl	Charlie Schicht
Debbie Ellis	Jack Schicht
Kim Exeler	Sandra Sims
Terry Foster	Kaira Simmons
Sarah Giolando	Benita Utz
Luke Groeschen	Janice Way

Foreword

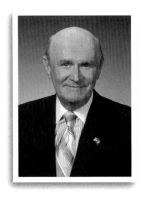

Dear Community,

Welcome to a special publication commemorating St. Elizabeth Health-care's 150-year history. We have a proud heritage of providing excellent care and devoted service to our community. For 150 years, we have been building upon a solid foundation of comprehensive and compassionate care that improves the health of the people we serve. St. Elizabeth Healthcare is not only the largest healthcare provider in Northern Kentucky, but is also continually recognized as one of the nation's best.

As we celebrate the accomplishments of the past, we look ahead to what we will accomplish for the future. Within our thriving, multi-faceted organization, we have some of the nation's top medical professionals work-ing together to guarantee the best care is delivered for generations to come.

We thank all of the wonderful and generous people who have support-ed St. Elizabeth Healthcare over our remarkable history. We look forward with great excitement and anticipation to implementing new and innovative ways to deliver seamless care that ensures our patients and community will have access to the very best care and treatment spanning another 150 years and beyond.

We hope our 150th Anniversary book will inspire you as it continues to inspire us.

Sincerely,

Michael J. Gibbons
Chairman, Board of Trustees
St. Elizabeth Healthcare

Introduction

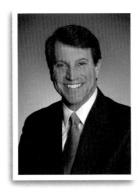

Dear Friends,

On January 21, 1861, just three months before the first shot of the Civil War was fired, St. Elizabeth opened its doors on Seventh Street in Covington with 10 patient beds. Today, St. Elizabeth Healthcare has six major facilities stretching across five Northern Kentucky counties and we are the area's largest employer, with more than 7,300 associates. For 150 years, St. Elizabeth Healthcare has been the heart and soul of healthcare in Northern Kentucky. Over that time, we have grown into the topnotch, multi-faceted organization that all of Greater Cincinnati views today as the gold standard in medicine.

St. Elizabeth's growth has remained as steady and firm-footed as our mission. From our humble beginnings to the present, St. Elizabeth has never wavered from our mission of improving the health and well-being of those we are so privileged to serve. St. Elizabeth Healthcare has a strong history of excellence and continues to offer an unparalleled level of expertise in an environment of unending compassion, while growing in both quality and scope of services for care.

This anniversary book honors the spirit of our founders whose vision to care for the less fortunate has grown substantially and touched so many lives in the process. Today, we stand with them, looking forward to building a future that others will be proud to build upon as well.

Enjoy your journey through these pages as you experience the rich, vibrant history and current life of St. Elizabeth Healthcare that has taken 150 memorable years to create. The snapshots of St. Elizabeth's history will tell a story of an organization whose level of care and strength has nurtured the growth and health of the entire Northern Kentucky region. While we reminisce on our past, we can continue to look forward to our next 150 years.

Sincerely,

John S. Dubis, FACHE
President & Chief Executive Officer
St. Elizabeth Healthcare

Chapter 1

The Princess, the Crusader, the Sparrow and the Scholar

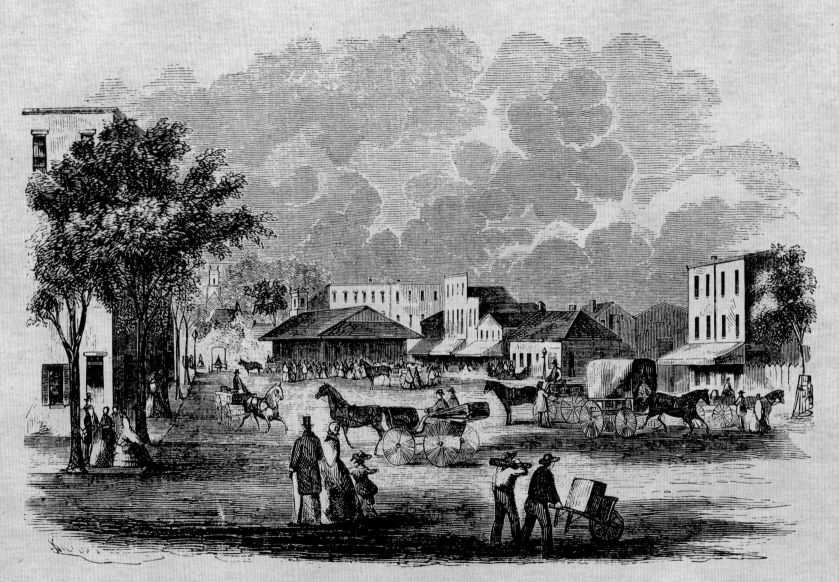

MARKET AND SQUARE, COVINGTON, KY.

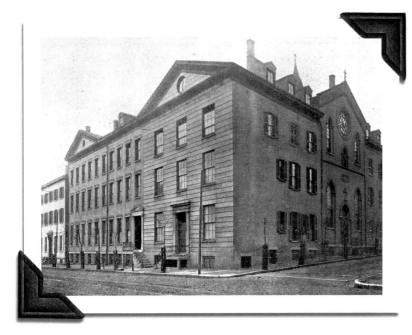

Sarah Worthington King Peter turned her mansion at Third and Lytle Streets over to the Sisters of the Poor of St. Francis. From: *Souvenir Album of American Cities: Catholic Churches of Cincinnati and Hamilton County, Ohio* (Cincinnati, 1896).

Opposite: Sarah Worthington King Peter (1800–1877), daughter of American political leader Thomas Worthington, played an important role in the founding of St. Elizabeth Hospital. From: Anna Shannon McAllister, *In Winter We Flourish: Life and Letters of Sarah Peter* (New York: Longmans, Green and Co., 1939).

Previous page: City of Covington, Market and Square, much as it would have looked when St. Elizabeth Hospital opened in 1861. From: *Ballou's Pictorial Drawing Room Companion,* December 20, 1856.

The founding of St. Elizabeth Hospital is the account of remarkable people achieving overwhelming goals in challenging and contentious times. The United States was at a crossroads, torn apart by divisions of politics, culture, economics, geography and race. Nearly 10 percent of the nation's population was held in bondage, and about one-third of the nation was willing to take up arms against the rest of the country, defending with blood and bullet what they perceived as their God-given rights. No one was sure whether this young experiment in democracy would survive to see its glorious first centennial, or whether the nation would settle into anarchy and chaos, divided into smaller nations separated by culture, politics and a brutal Civil War.

Nowhere was this division more evident than in the Northern Kentucky-Cincinnati region. One side of the great Ohio River was free from slavery, a beacon for those who sought to make their way out of bondage. The other side, equally diverse, still featured human bondage. In 1860, the tension between the two sides of the river must have been palpable.

It was during this time of great upheaval and uncertainty that a group of visionaries worked together to create St. Elizabeth Hospital. The hospital symbolized how human needs and suffering transcends the immediate cares of the world. These remarkable people were stating to a chaotic world that life would continue, and that what they sought to build would furnish hope for a better tomorrow. As one nun said during the founding of the second St. Elizabeth Hospital on 11th Street in 1867, "The new hospital will not only be an ornament to the City of Covington, but a blessing for centuries."[1]

"A blessing for centuries": A hope, a wish or a promise? One may wonder what the founders of the hospital would think of St. Elizabeth today, with its six hospitals and numerous health centers. They probably would not be surprised because they were people of vision. Each in their own way had seen the best and the worst of life, and chose, individually, to make life better for others. The visionaries behind the founding of the St. Elizabeth hospital include Sarah Worthington King Peter, Henrietta Esther Scott Cleveland, Sister Frances Schervier and Bishop George Aloysius Carrell.

The Princess

If the state of Ohio had a royal family it would be the Worthingtons. Thomas Worthington, often called by historians "the father of Ohio statehood," was Ohio's first United States senator and its sixth

governor. He is given credit for negotiating the Ohio territory into the Union as America's 17th state; he was friends with Thomas Jefferson, James Madison and Aaron Burr. The great seal of the state of Ohio was literally drawn based on the view from the front porch of his estate, called Adena. In short, Thomas Worthington was an important player in early America. As a result, his children, including his daughter Sarah, grew up among some of the most important people of the time.

Being a child of such prestigious birth did not guarantee a life of luxury without suffering. Sarah's sister Mary married David Macomb, a handsome man from an important family. Macomb was a ne'er-do-well and quickly gambled away his wife's money. Thomas Worthington attempted to help his daughter and son-in-law by giving the young family a mill to manage and a fine home on Paint Creek near Chillicothe, Ohio. Unfortunately, Macomb continued his bad habits and soon fled Ohio with his wife and young family to Texas, where he believed he could avoid his debts. In Texas,

without the support of his wealthy father-in-law, matters grew worse and soon Macomb and his family were once again in trouble. In 1836, Mary died and soon after Macomb committed suicide by cutting his throat, leaving the children destitute.

Sarah Worthington's life was not much better than that of her sister. Sarah's first husband, Edward King, was also handsome but troubled by gambling. Like his father-in-law, King was active in politics and served in the Ohio legislature. Once, while Edward was away in Columbus attending a session of the legislature, the Ross County sheriff came to Sarah's home and notified her that she and her family soon would be evicted from their home in order to repay her husband's debts. The family, with considerable help from Thomas Worthington, was able to pay the debts, but they were forced to sell their home. They lived in a rental house for the remainder of their life together in Chillicothe. In 1836, Edward King died, leaving his young wife with a mountain of debt and two sons to raise.

Sarah wanted to further her education, but the subjects she wanted to pursue were not considered appropriate for women. When her sons attended Harvard College, she went along to serve as a housemother for them and her nephews. The arrangement saved money, but she found it somewhat embarrassing. While at Harvard, Sarah took advantage of the learning environment, hiring tutors to teach subjects she found interesting. Her second marriage to a much older man, William Peter, was the direct result of a desire not to become a financial burden to her sons. The marriage was not a happy one, but being a woman in a man's world, Sarah's choices were limited.[2] Perhaps it was her hardships and those of her sister that inspired her lifelong concern for women and children.

In 1854, Sarah converted to Catholicism. The Catholic Church offered not only a way to salvation, but also a means to intervene on behalf of women, children and the poor. The Catholic religious orders that Worthington encountered during her travels, especially in Europe, seemed above politics, governments or the changes in society that often brought turmoil and upheaval. Their concerns were for those who had little choice and few options in life. They genuinely cared for others, and Sarah Worthington King Peter found this refreshing.

Worthington was influential in the creation of St. Mary's Hospital in Cincinnati, Ohio, in 1858. She had convinced the Archbishop of Cincinnati to allow her to travel to Europe, to persuade a group of nuns to immigrate to America to start a hospital. This made Worthington an ideal choice to help establish a hospital in Northern Kentucky. She had vision, desire and had now done this before.

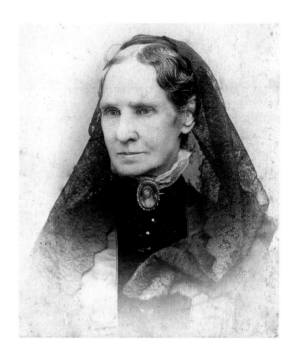

The Crusader

Henrietta Esther Scott Cleveland came from tough American pioneer stock. Her maternal grandfather was Major Jacob Fowler, one of the first settlers in the Northern Kentucky region. He surveyed roads, built the first log cabin in Newport, operated a ferry on the Licking River and nearly died fighting Indians at St. Clair's Defeat in the Ohio country. He took part in the Battle of Fallen Timbers, served in the War of 1812 and, in 1821 at the age of 57, was hired by the federal government to survey the upper Arkansas River. In 1844, at the age of 80, he was described as being as young and vigorous as a man 30 years his

---

2 Correspondence with Pat Medert, curator, Ross County Historical Society, September 7, 2010. The Ross County Historical Society is the repository of the Sarah Worthington King Peter Papers.

junior, with no gray hair and the ability to shoot a squirrel at 100 yards with ease.[3]

Major Fowler's daughter, Abigail, married Major Chasteen Scott, who also served his country in the War of 1812. The Scott family was related by marriage not only to the Fowler family, but also to the families

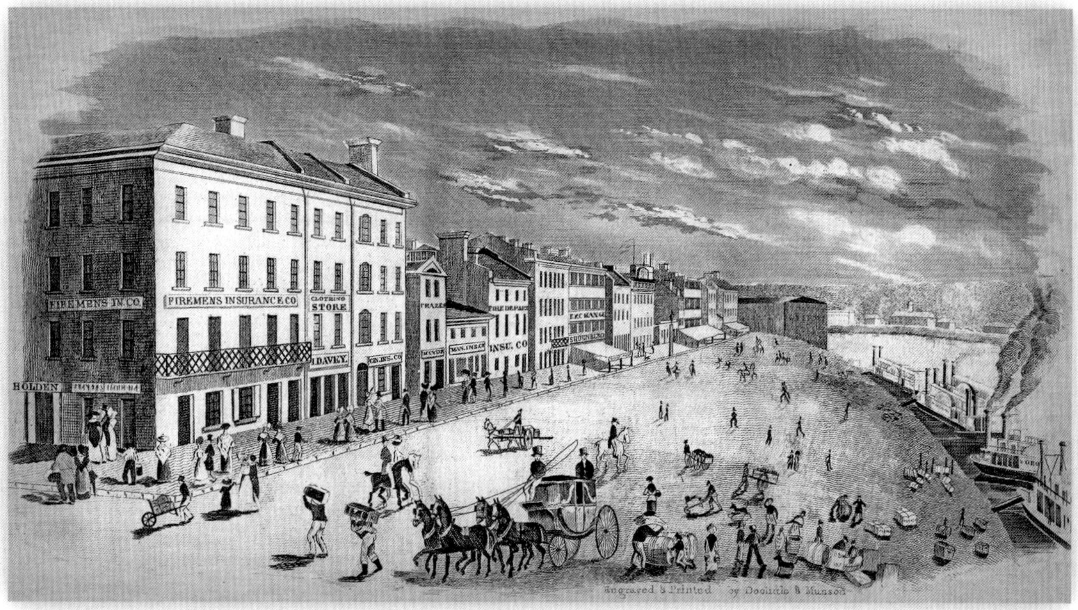

of John Cleves Symmes and President William Henry Harrison. The Scotts and the Fowlers owned large farms in Boone County, Kentucky, along Fowler Creek, as well as property in the city of Covington. In 1834, Henrietta Scott, the daughter of Chasteen and Abigail, married George P. Cleveland, son of Rev. Charles Cleveland. In 1816, Rev. Cleveland founded the Boston Society for the Moral and Religious Instruction of the Poor. Young George was 8 years old when his father founded the society, perhaps influencing the young Cleveland's interest in charitable work.

In 1836, George and Henrietta Cleveland gave birth to a son, Charles, presumably named after George's father. Sadly, the child died just two years later. The following year, 1839, the young couple purchased from Henrietta's father a drug store called the Black Mortar on Covington's Market Space. Less than a year later, George Cleveland died at age 31, leaving his widow, Henrietta, one month pregnant with a second son.[4]

Henrietta returned to the home of her father, and when her son George was old enough, he was sent to St. Xavier College in Cincinnati (now Xavier University). Colleges at that time usually operated preparatory schools which accepted young scholars. Perhaps it was sometime during this period of living with her father that Henrietta converted to Catholicism. During the summer of 1851, two events took place that

Bidenharn, Wm. T., do
Bamber, Henry,... do
Camp, Robert,....New Orleans.
Carcaut, John,....Louisiana.
Cleveland, George,.Kentucky.
Claverie, Alcide,..Louisiana.
Coyne, Nicholas J.,Ohio.
Campbell, Philip,.Wheeling, Va.
Drummond, H.,...Alabama.
Drummond, Th.,.. do
Dietrich, Charles,..Cincinnati.
Doumeing, Emile,.Louisiana.

would change Henrietta forever. On July 8, 1851, George died at the age of 11. That same summer, George Aloysius Carrell came to Cincinnati to become the head of St. Xavier College. There is little doubt that the death of the young George Cleveland brought Henrietta and the future Bishop

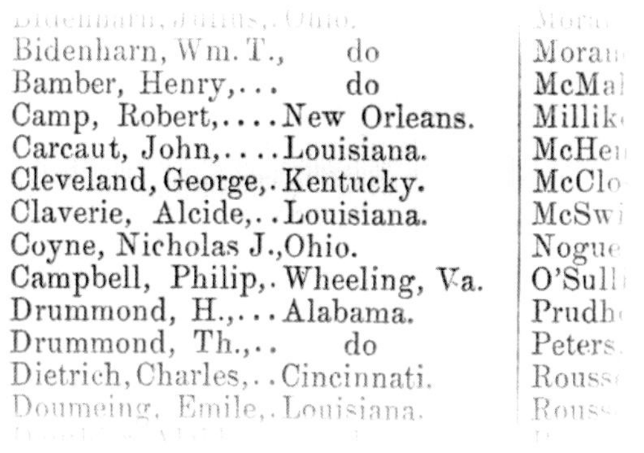

3 Tenkotte, Paul, A., David E. Schroeder, and Thomas Ward, *To Be Catholic and American in Northern, Central and Appalachian Kentucky: The Diocese of Covington, 1853–2003* (unpublished manuscript in possession of the author) and Jacob Fowler: 1764–1849, accessed at *www.rootsweb.ancestry.com/~kycampbe/jacobfowler.htm* on December 29, 2010.

4 Tenkotte, Paul, A., David E. Schroeder, and Thomas Ward, *To Be Catholic and American in Northern, Central and Appalachian Kentucky: The Diocese of Covington, 1853–2003* (unpublished manuscript in possession of the author), p. 46.

of Covington together for the first time, which cemented a relationship that would help establish the founding of St. Elizabeth Hospital.

Henrietta Scott Cleveland seems to have taken the death of her son as a call to action. She became active in the Catholic Church, even helping to sew the religious vestments for George Carrell when he was named Bishop of Covington in 1853.[5] She became president of the Ladies Society of Covington, which focused the leading women of the community in efforts on behalf of the poor. In addition to this work, Cleveland visited the families of the poor and those in distress and did what she could to make the lives of the impoverished more tolerable. It was probably during these visits that she became acutely aware of the needs of the growing Northern Kentucky community, including the necessity for a hospital. She was certain that Covington needed a hospital, so she became relentless in the pursuit of the project, never once surrendering to the overwhelming odds against her. Like her ancestral pioneer stock, Henrietta Scott Cleveland always moved forward—seldom looking backwards—for a cause she knew was right.

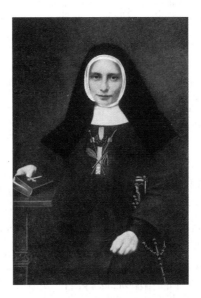

Sr. Frances Schervier (1819–1876), founder of the Sisters of Poor of St. Francis, who staffed the first St. Elizabeth Hospital. From: St. Elizabeth Healthcare.

Opposite:

Newport and Covington Suspension Bridge. From: *Ballou's Pictorial Drawing Room Companion*, December 20, 1856.

5 Tenkotte, Paul, A., David E. Schroeder, and Thomas Ward, *To Be Catholic and American in Northern, Central and Appalachian Kentucky: The Diocese of Covington, 1853–2003* (unpublished manuscript in possession of the author), p, 46.

The Sparrow

The world into which Frances Schervier was born was one of alarming contrasts. The city of Aachen had been occupied by France, but was part of a yet-to-be-unified Germany. Most of the people living in the city found both their language and mannerisms coming from France, including Frances' mother, Marie Louise Schervier. The city had long been in the international spotlight, ever since it served as the capital of Charlemagne's Holy Roman Empire. In addition, Aachen was a major industrial center boasting a number of important industries, one of which was a pin factory owned by Frances' father.

Yet with all these advantages, the great city of Aachen was backward, both socially and politically. The advantages of being a multi-cultural city, constantly in the center of what was going on in Europe, did not filter down to most of its inhabitants. The city was a study in contrast between the rich and the poor. Aachen had some of the best minds and most influential politicians of the era, but the city itself still held onto its almost medieval form of government and economic system. The result was a community slow to change and modernize, leaving many of its people to suffer from overcrowding, poor sanitation and ever decreasing economic opportunity.

Frances Schervier was born on January 3, 1819. Her mother was French and her father was German. Her parents were both Catholic, but not active in the church. According to one of Frances Schervier's biographers, Petra Fietzek, the young Frances was greatly influenced by one of her teachers, Luise Hensel. Hensel was a deeply religious woman who helped Frances make sense of the conflicting world around her. Hensel taught her students to act on behalf of the poor and suffering whom they saw throughout the city. Her influence on the children greatly concerned their parents, who eventually worked to have Hensel removed from the school. One of the signers of the petition to remove Luise Hensel was Johann Heinrich Schervier, Frances' father.[6]

At age 8, Frances had a dream that would influence her for the rest of her life. In her dream, Frances was called by the principal of the school to meet a man who had come to see her. The man was Jesus, and he took her into his arms. She felt a love that she had never felt before. She then realized that this love she felt was what people have described as unconditional love. To Frances, Jesus was only asking for her love in return, which would be manifested in doing his work among the people who needed it most.[7] To her, Jesus' words "Unto the least of these my brethren you have done unto me…" had real meaning as a call to service.[8]

As Frances grew older, she became more and more devout, a fact that concerned her parents greatly. Her father's greatest fear and often stated complaint was that someday she might join a convent. Her father's fear may have been somewhat justified. Although a Catholic himself, he was not active in the faith. As a well-connected businessman and local politician, he may have been aware of the anti-Catholic feelings that were beginning to grow in the country. Having a child so close to a church that was falling into disfavor may have been troubling to Johann Schervier. Nonetheless, despite her father's objections, Frances labored on, both in her faith and in her service to the poor.

At the tender age of 12, Frances learned firsthand about the differences between the rich and the poor in her community. In 1830 a workers' riot broke out in Aachen, resulting in considerable property damage and loss of life. The workers protested the introduction of mechanized steam power

---

8 Book of Mathew, Revised Standard Version.

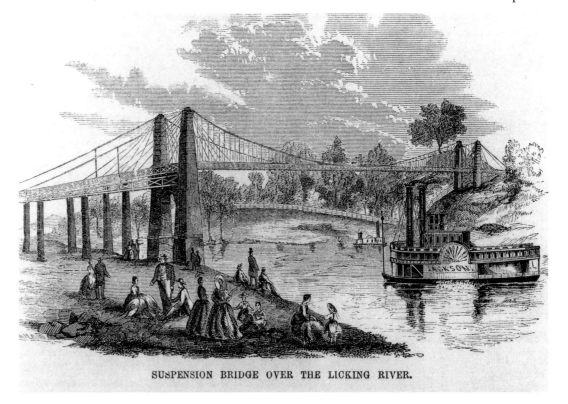

SUSPENSION BRIDGE OVER THE LICKING RIVER.

---

6 Fietzek, Petra. *The Life of Frances Schervier: Words are Not Enough*, 2002 , Sisters of the Poor of St. Francis, Aachen, Germany, p. 9.

7 Fietzek, p. 9.

and machinery in the factories, as well as unfair and unsafe working conditions for women and children.[9] New technologies did away with skilled labor, forcing wages down and eliminating jobs. Frustrated, workers felt they had no choice, but to take to the streets. The riot was violently suppressed by soldiers and armed members of the community.

The Catholic Church worked to calm tension in the city by acting as an intermediary between workers and factory owners. One such factory owner, a man named Fay, worked with a local priest to help create a dialogue with his workers. Fay's daughter was a schoolmate of Frances', who was eager to hear of the work of the priest.[10] It was yet another example to Frances that the church had an important role in healing a troubled people. A few years later, when epidemics of cholera and tuberculosis ravaged the city and even took the life of her beloved mother, Frances again witnessed the power of good people reaching out in the name of God to help others.

Frances volunteered to work in her parish's soup kitchen. She actively helped with a young priest, Father Johann Istas, to build the kitchen and collect food and supplies to give to the poor. She led the soup kitchen after the death of the young priest.

Meanwhile, Frances talked openly to trusted family members and priests about joining a religious order. She was told about the work and calling of St. Francis of Assisi to serve the poor and live simply.

In 1844, Frances could not wait any longer. The call of God to serve was too great so Frances joined the secular Third Order of St. Francis. However, joining this group was still not enough for Frances. Later that same year a friend reported to her that she had a message for Frances from Jesus. Jesus had told her that Frances must commit herself to Christ fully and heal the wounds of his people.[11] Frances was torn, but convinced that the call was genuine. She questioned the source, a devout friend, but felt the calling deep in her heart and soul. After much consideration, she and several women established the Sisters of the Poor of St. Francis in a rented house in Aachen.

Despite what seemed a reluctant start, Frances embraced her new life with enthusiasm and bravery. She was quickly elected Mother Superior by her fellow sisters. She and her small order immediately began to work with the poorest of the poor and those people that society had turned their backs against. One of the main efforts of the small group was to help the many prostitutes and "fallen women" who currently occupied the town. Sister Frances was not above dressing as a man to rescue prostitutes from local brothels. She did what it took to meet the needs of the people she served. It was a trait that her fellow sisters learned well, and soon the tiny order of nuns had a reputation for doing so much with so little, especially with the poor and the sick.

Frances likened herself and her fellow sisters to sparrows. Sparrows are small, brown, unassuming birds that spend their days joyfully singing, busily building their nests and gathering food. The culture created by Sister Frances in her small convent was one of constant joy in the face of difficult hardships. Each challenge or misfortune was an opportunity to show the power of God and of divine blessings.

It is therefore no surprise that when Sarah Worthington King Peter came looking for an order of nuns to open the first Catholic hospital in Cincinnati, she was sent to Frances Schervier and her small congregation of sisters. After a long discussion with Sarah Peter, Sister Schervier somewhat reluctantly sent three of her nuns to the United States. Three years later in 1861, Sister Schervier was approached again to send three of her fellow sisters to America for another new hospital to be located in Covington, Kentucky. This time Sister Schervier sent three sisters, Antonia, Stylita and Joachim, and apostulant, Susanna Oechner. Like the sparrows, these three sisters, unfamiliar with America, went cheerfully on this journey to a new nation, ready to meet the challenges.

9 "Aachen History," accessed at *www.aachen.de/EN/ts/160_about_aachen/20_aachen_history/index.html* on November 8, 2010.

10 Fietzek, p. 10.

11 Fietzek, p. 32.

The Scholar

When Bishop Carrell died in 1868, his funeral procession was nearly a mile long.[12] It was comprised of members of his Catholic flock, school children, members of religious orders, important dignitaries from nearby dioceses and many non-Catholic civic and community leaders. Overall it was a grand affair, fitting the status of a man who had spearheaded the establishment of the Catholic Diocese of Covington.

12 *Covington Journal*, October 3, 1868.

George Aloysius Carrell was loved and respected by both his congregation and his civic peers. However, this was not the life that he would have chosen for himself. The life that Carrell longed for was a quieter, more scholarly life, shaping the minds and futures of eager students. The life of an educator is what Carrell really wanted, a dream he kept alive throughout his career as Bishop of Covington. Some would argue that it was his eventual surrender of that dream that ended his life.

Before being selected by Pope Pius IX to become the first bishop of the new Diocese of Covington, the Rev. George Carrell was the director of St. Xavier Preparatory School, which eventually became Xavier University in Cincinnati. George Carrell was born in Philadelphia, Pennsylvania in 1808, the son of John and Mary Carrell. John Carrell is listed in the 1785 Philadelphia Directory as being a goldsmith and watchmaker. He was a strong supporter of the Catholic Church in Philadelphia, serving a number of church leadership roles. George's grandfather, Timothy, an Irish immigrant, was a successful wine merchant and grocer who pledged generously in 1762 to the building fund of St. Mary's Catholic Church in Philadelphia.[13] St. Mary's played an important role in the history of the American Colonial period and the American Revolution. Famous worshipers who attended services at St. Mary's included George Washington and John Adams, as well as many members of the Continental Congress when America's capital city was Philadelphia.[14]

13 Records of the American Catholic Historical Society of Philadelphia, vol. 15, p. 402.

14 "Old St. Mary's Church & Cemetery," accessed at *www.ushistory.org/tour/st.marys.htm* on December 24, 2010.

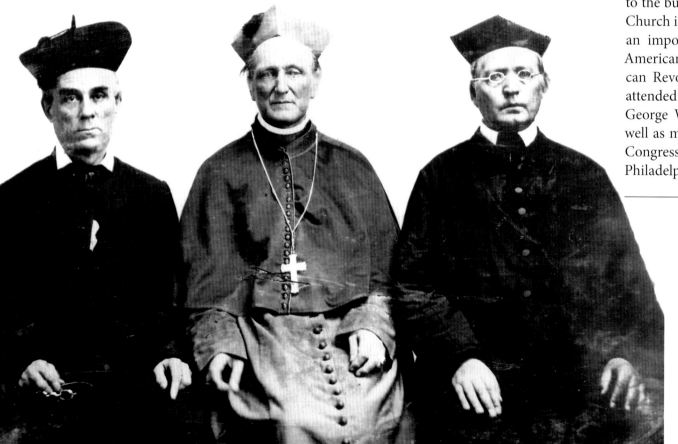

Left to right: Rev. Thomas Butler (1836–1869); Roman Catholic Bishop George Carrell (1803–1868); and Rev. Ferdinand Kühr (1806–1870). Carrell served as bishop of Covington during the founding of St. Elizabeth Hospital. From: Archives of the Diocese of Covington.

The home where Bishop Carrell was born and raised was a large yet simple mansion that once belonged to William Penn. Penn, a prominent leader in the Quaker Church, had used his influence and financial recourses to establish the Quaker Colony of Pennsylvania in 1681. Penn's colony was unique among the original 13 colonies because of its commitment to the fair treatment of immigrants and Indians living within the boundaries of the colony. Because of this fair treatment, which was based on Quaker principles, Pennsylvania became known as the "the best poor man's country."[15]

Perhaps it was these influences that helped shape Bishop Carrell's devotion to the poor and his desire to serve others. In 1827, Carrell was ordained a priest and in 1835, he joined the Society of Jesus (Jesuits). In 1843, he was named president of St. Louis University at a critical time in the institution's development. In 1842, the university had opened its medical school and in 1843 it began enrolling students for its new law school. Carrell remained president of the college until 1843 when he was appointed president of St. Xavier in Cincinnati.

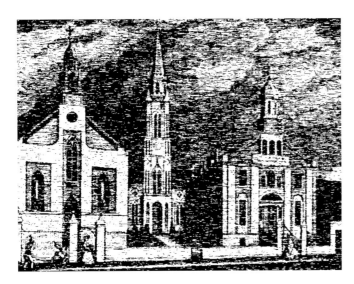

St. Xavier College, Cincinnati, where Bishop Carrell had served as president. From: St. Xavier College Catalogue (1850).

On July 29, 1853, George Aloysius Carrell was appointed the first Bishop of Covington. The newly created diocese had a grand total of six priests, 10 churches and little money. The position was one that Carrell would not have chosen for himself, but as a servant of the Lord, he went where he was called.

As the leader of Northern Kentucky's Catholic faith, Carrell was involved in all aspects of his diocese. He oversaw the building of churches, including the erection of St. Mary's Cathedral in 1854. He helped establish schools for both boys and girls, and supported many efforts on behalf of the poor. When it came to supporting the creation of St. Elizabeth Hospital, he held nothing back. The nuns at the hospital reported that they often found the Bishop personally inspecting the hospital's pantry looking for deficiencies. Shortfalls in fuel, milk or other necessaries would often be made up out of his own meager resources.[16] He took special interest in the Union soldiers who were placed at the hospital during the fall of 1862 and saw to it that they received everything they needed.

The American Civil War brought particular anguish to Bishop Carrell. The war that tore apart a nation caused heartache for the Catholic Church too. Despite a declaration by American bishops at the Third Provincial Council at Cincinnati in April of 1861 that there is "no north, no south, no east and no west," Catholic leadership

15 See Lemon, James T. *The Best Poor Man's Country: A Geographical Study of Early Southeastern Pennsylvania.* Baltimore: Johns Hopkins Press, 1972.

16 *History of St. Elizabeth Hospital, Covington, Kentucky, Under the Direction of the Sisters of the Poor of St. Francis from 1860-1880,* pp. 13-14.

was divided.[17] Bishop Carrell eliminated the *Catholic Telegraph* as his official newspaper because of its controversial political stands.[18] Carrell may have been conflicted, as many Americans were at the time. His grandfather had owned slaves and Kentucky was a slave state, yet his concern for all people would have made the practice of slave owning repugnant.[19] What seems to have bothered the Bishop most of all was the idea of conflict. When the news from the war front became too much for him, he requested that his subordinates give him no more.

Some, including the sisters of the hospital, claimed that Bishop Carrell died of a broken heart. He had spent his entire career as Bishop of Covington trying to keep the diocese running despite the Civil War and economic crisis. He was a man of deep feeling and commitment to the causes of his flock and to the poor of his community. He quite literally felt the pain of his people. A large motivator to keep him going was the hope that one day he would return to the life of an educator. This personal dream was manifested in the land that he purchased south of Covington (in present-day Fort Mitchell) where he opened the Preparatory College of St. Aloysius. Less than a year later, in January 1868, the bishop sold the seminary building and property to the St. John's Orphan Society.[20] The sisters at St. Elizabeth Hospital reported that the closing of his preparatory college broke the Bishop in both body and spirit. He passed away shortly thereafter, in September 1868.

17 Hennesey, James. *American Catholics: A History of the Roman Catholic Community in the United States*, (Oxford: Oxford University Press, 1981), p 153.

18 Hennesey, James. *American Catholics*, p 153, and McGreevy, John T. *Catholicism and American Freedom: A History*. (New York: W. W. Norton & Company, 2003), p. 82.

19 Records of the American Catholic Historical Society of Philadelphia, vol. 15 p. 402, records the baptism of one of Timothy Carrell's slaves.

20 Deed Book 38 (1866–1868), pp. 557–559, Kenton County Courthouse, Independence, Ky.

Rheumatism Cure 1860

Please do not try this at home

In addition to the medicines given under the head Rheumatic Fever, the most decided benefit can be derived from Alcoholic Vapor Baths, which, while they will not in the least interfere with the actions of the medicines, tend greatly to

"Then set fire to the alcohol and if the heat is too great, raise the edge of the blanket and let it be reduced. Continue this until he sweats freely, or becomes too much fatigued to sit longer."

mitigate the pains, and produce an equal state of circulation by stimulating the surface; abridging in many cases, the disease one-half the time it would run under the long interval treatment alone. This treatment is to be applied by filling a tea cup full of alcohol, placed in a saucer of water to insure against danger from an overflow while burning. Place both under a solid wood bottom seat chair, elevated about the thickness of a brick under each post, strip the patient naked and give him an alkaline bath, and rubbing his surface dry, place him upon the chair, enveloping him completely, except his head, with a woolen sheet or blanket, (as there is no danger of the wool taking fire,) letting the blanket enclose also the chair and come to the floor. Then set fire to the alcohol and if the heat is too great, raise the edge of the blanket and let it be reduced. Continue this until he sweats freely, or becomes too much fatigued to sit longer. Let the patient often drink freely of cold water during the process. Remove him from the chair to his bed and cover him warmly. It is well to place the feet in hot water during the process. This is a delightful operation for the rheumatic patient, and no one will object to a repetition of it. Whatever physicians may think or say of this operation, I know it is a most potent agent for the cure of inflammatory rheumatism, and is a valuable agent in the chronic form of the disease.

An Epitome of the Homeopathic Healing Art, Containing the New Discoveries and Improvements to the Present Time; Designed for the use of Families and Travelers and as a Pocket Companion for the Physician, 11th Edition, by B. L. Hill, M.D. (Professor of General, Special and Surgical Anatomy, late Professor of Surgery, Obstetrics, and Diseases of Women and Children, in the W.H. College, Author of the "Homeopathic Practice of Surgery" & c., & c., 1864. (pages 27–28)

Chapter 2

The First St. Elizabeth

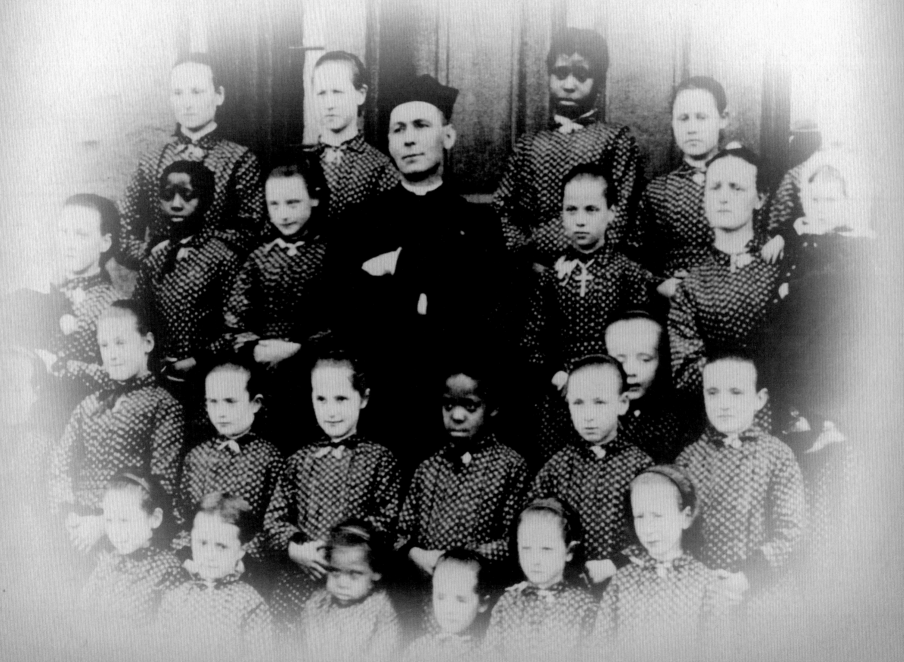

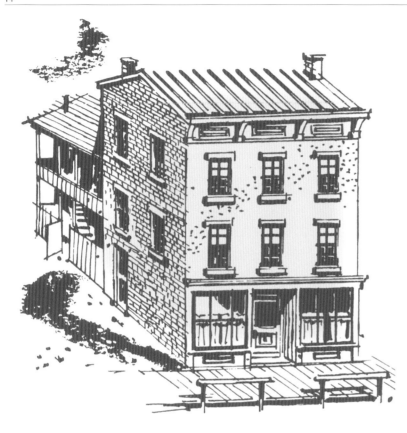

The first building of St. Elizabeth Hospital, 7th St., Covington. From: One Hundred Twenty-Five Years: St. Elizabeth Medical Center (1986).

Opposite: The 1877 City Atlas of Covington shows the first location of St. Elizabeth Hospital, on the south side of 7th Street, between Madison and Scott Sts. The lot is identified as owned by Bishop Carroll [sic], although he died in 1868. From: City Atlas of Covington, Kentucky (C. M. Hopkins, 1877).

Previous page: St. Elizabeth Foundling Asylum cared for children of all ages and races. From: Archives of the Diocese of Covington.

"We are about to have a hospital in our midst."[1] With these words the *Covington Journal* announced to the people of Northern Kentucky that they soon would have a hospital, calling it an answer to "one of the wants of our city."[2] The paper further went on to state, for those worried that a new hospital would bring unwanted and contagious illnesses into the city, that "no persons suffering from contagious diseases would be admitted" to the new hospital.

Keeping those with contagious diseases out of the hospital was probably the least of the worries which the founders of the hospital had on their minds. A lot of hard work had to take place long before any patients of any kind would be admitted. Not the least of the concerns of the founders was finding a suitable location for the hospital and convincing Bishop Carrell of the Diocese of Covington that the first hospital should be operated by the Catholic Church.

In 1858, Sarah Worthington King Peter convinced the Archbishop of Cincinnati, John Baptist Purcell, that the city needed a Catholic hospital to "care for the destitute poor of German nationality" in the city.[3] The Archbishop granted permission for Peter to travel to Europe and to consult with the Vatican on the matter.

1 Covington Journal, November 24, 1860.

2 Covington Journal, November 24, 1860.

3 "Sisters of the Poor" from the Catholic Encyclopedia, accessed at *www.newadvent.org/cathen/12257a.htm* on October 27, 2010.

She was even granted an audience with the Pope. Peter was told, while visiting Rome, that she should "go find some willing German nuns" to immigrate to America to start a new order and to establish a hospital in Cincinnati.[4] Peter found a willing order of nuns, the Sisters of the Poor of St. Francis, headed by Frances Schervier.

At the time, the Sisters of the Poor of St. Francis were a small order of nuns with the reputation of helping the poorest of the poor, especially those people whom other caregivers often shunned. This group included individuals with communicable diseases like tuberculosis and social diseases like syphilis. The reputation of the sisters as nurses was remarkable.

Founded by Sister Schervier in 1845, the small order had grown to only 23 sisters by 1851.[5] By the time of Sarah Peter's visit in March 1858, the small order numbered about 45. Peter was impressed with what she found—hard-working nuns, a clean and orderly house, and people in need being served. She reported in a letter to friends that "I know of no Order which does as much as this."[6] Furthermore, Sister Schervier and Peter hit it off well and de-

veloped a genuine rapport with each other. Sister Schervier agreed to send five nuns and a postulant across the ocean to Cincinnati to establish a branch of the order and a hospital there. The hospital they founded on the north side of the river was St. Mary's.

In early 1860, Chasteen Scott was preparing his will. As the patriarch of a significant Northern Kentucky family he had a number of affairs to settle. Something had to be done about his farms, his enslaved human property and his considerable property holdings in the city of Covington.[7] Most of his Covington property would go to his daughter Henrietta Cleveland. She

---

4 McAllister, Anna Shannon, *In Winter We Flourish: Life and Letters of Sarah Worthington King Peter* (New York: Longmans, Green and Company, 1939), pp. 263–264.

5 McAllister, Anna Shannon, *In Winter We Flourish: Life and Letters of Sarah Worthington King Peter, 1800–1877,* (New York: Longmans, Green and Company, 1939), p. 284.

6 McAllister, Anna Shannon, *In Winter We Flourish,* p. 284.

7 Unpublished will of Chasteen Scott, June 21, 1860, accessed at *files.usgwarchives.org/ky/kenton/wills /s2300002.txt.*

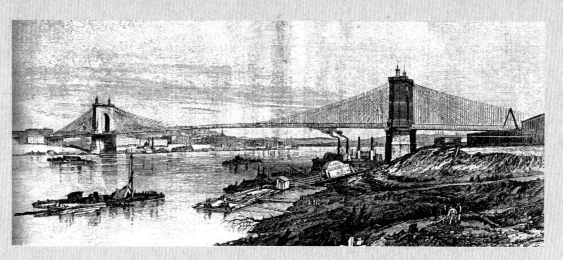

John Roebling's Covington and Cincinnati Suspension Bridge. From: *Frank Leslie's Illustrated Newspaper*, August 17, 1867.

was to inherit buildings, businesses and vacant land, but no slaves, perhaps because her conversion to Catholicism made the ownership of humans offensive to her. One way or another, in the summer of 1860 Cleveland found herself on the verge of an inheritance that would give her a sizeable portion of the city of Covington. The city in 1860 was beginning to come into its own. It boasted a number of mills, a glass factory, a brass foundry, two female academies, two weekly newspapers and a growing population of about 14,000 people.[8] Many of these residents were new arrivals, who had come either as single men or with their families, eager to find work in the growing city. The population of the county had grown by nearly 50 percent between 1850 and 1860. Nearly half of the new arrivals were born outside the United States.[9] Because of the city's rapid growth, housing for the new arrivals was often difficult to come by, forcing many to find temporary shelter

in overcrowded boarding houses near the riverfront.

As a result of this rapid growth, community services and sanitation were stretched to capacity and beyond. Communicable diseases like cholera and tuberculosis were common in the community, brought by the river commerce and the many poor who flocked to the city looking for opportunity. Traditionally, ill people counted on friends and family to care for them, but many of the new arrivals who now made Covington their home did not have this luxury. The hardships were even more difficult for those who were single, especially women, because of the confines of Victorian modesty. People without the benefit of family nearby or those living in overcrowded housing would have to seek help elsewhere, such as a kindly neighbor or a local hospital. In 1860 Covington had no hospital.

Perhaps this was the inspiration that motivated Henrietta Cleveland. Seeing the needs that the growing community was facing, combined with the fact that she was about to become a major property owner in the city, increased her feeling of responsibility to do something for her community. Cleveland was a woman of action and she could not wait for the city fathers to move forward on the subject; there had already been enough talk.

Cleveland knew that the best chance of getting a hospital that would meet the needs of the diverse people of Covington was through the Catholic Church. Her first conversation was with the head of the Diocese of Covington, Bishop George Aloysius Carrell. Carrell, although supportive of the idea, was not convinced that a hospital project could be accomplished by the diocese. The need was there, the Bishop would have freely admitted, as his love for the

8 Hawes, George W., Kentucky State Gazetteer and Business Directory for 1859 and 1860, accessed at *www.nkyviews.com* (Northern Kentucky Views) on November 10, 2010.

9 United States Census for Kenton County, Kentucky, 1850 and 1860. University of Virginia Library, Historical Census Browser, accessed at *mapserver.lib.virginia.edu/php/county.php* on November 10, 2010.

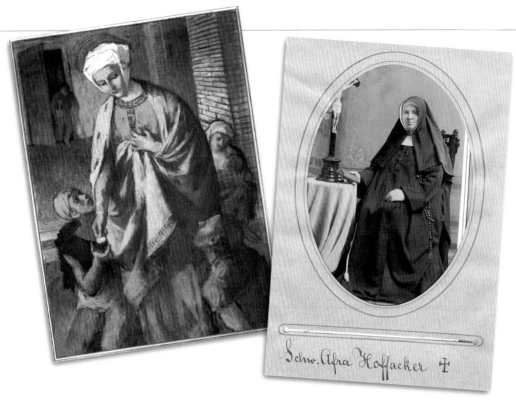

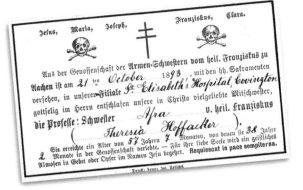

in local newspapers. It was decided by the sisters that the hospital would be named after St. Elizabeth of Hungary (1207–1231), who devoted her life to the poor and the sick. Elizabeth was the daughter of King Andrew II of Hungary, and was known for her charitable work with the poor and the sick. She lived during a time of political upheaval in her native land. Even her beloved mother was killed by political assassins. After the death of her husband, Ludwig IV, she joined the followers of St. Francis and devoted herself to charitable work, including founding a hospital. She died at age 24. Soon after her death a number of miraculous cures were reported, leading to her sainthood in 1235.[16] As a namesake for the new hospital in Covington, St. Elizabeth was a perfect choice, given her charitable work at a time of political unrest. On the verge of the Civil War, Northern Kentucky was likewise in need of acts of mercy.

As soon as the building was obtained, the sisters began work to get it ready for its first patients. Before the building could be made livable it needed a thorough cleaning. The sisters dedicated to this task boarded with sisters in Cincinnati. They were ferried every morning across the Ohio River to do their work at the new hospital building. With no heat in the building and no stove to heat the water that they used to clean with, the work must have been miserable. One sister reported that if she left her hand too long on a freshly washed wall, her hand would freeze to the wet wall. The sisters looked upon these hardships as a challenge to their commitment to God, which they accepted cheerfully.[17]

By mid-January the sisters had the hospital ready for its first patient. They did not have to wait long. On January 23, 1861, Dr.

---

16 "St. Elizabeth of Hungary," The Catholic Encyclopedia, accessed at *newadvent.org/cathen/05389a.htm*, on November 11, 2010.

17 *History of St. Elizabeth Hospital, Covington, Kentucky, Under the Direction of the Sisters of the Poor of St. Francis from 1860–1880*, pp. 13–15.

Joseph Schwarz sent St. Elizabeth Hospital its first patient. His name was Louis Myer (Meyer). He was 35 years old, a laborer, married with three young children, and he was dying. According to the 1860 census, the Myer family was living in an overcrowded boarding house in Covington's Sixth Ward. The family included his wife, Louisa, and his sons, Henry (9 years old), William (5 years old), and George (3 months old). Louis, Louisa and Henry had been born in Hannover, Germany, while William had been born in Ohio and young George in Kentucky, indicating that the family had moved often.[18]

The intake records of the hospital state that Myer suffered from "rheumatism," which may have manifested itself in painful incapacity. In some cases, the bones of the lower spine and pelvis become brittle causing them to break easily. If this were the case with Louis Myer, not only could he not work as a laborer and support his family, he also would be completely dependent on others for his basic needs. His wife could hardly have managed the care of her husband, let alone an infant and two young boys. St. Elizabeth Hospital would have been the best of the family's limited options.

As testimony to the sisters' commitment to help all those in need despite color, creed or religious background, St. Elizabeth Hospital's first patient was a Protestant. This fact did not matter to the sisters in the least, for he was a man in need; however, it did lead to at least one awkward moment for the Catholic nuns. Upon his arrival at the hospital, Louis Myer asked that a certain pastor come for a visitation. While there, he asked the minister to give him communion, which in some Protestant denominations is a symbolic act rather than a sacrament as it is to the Catholic faithful. After the completion of the communion service, the minister offered the leftover wine and bread to the postulant Susanna Oechner, who was probably shocked at the casual treatment of what she believed was sacred. She politely refused the minister's offering.[19]

Intake record showing St. Elizabeth Hospital's first patient, Louis Meyer, January 23, 1861. From: Kenton County Public Library, Covington.

Opposite: St. Elizabeth Foundling Asylum cared for children of all ages and races. From: Archives of the Diocese of Covington.

18 1860 United States Census for the City of Covington, Kentucky, Ward 6, microfilm roll M653-379, p. 855, image 573. Accessed through *Ancestry.com* on September 7, 2010.

19 *History of St. Elizabeth Hospital, Covington, Kentucky, Under the Direction of the Sisters of the Poor of St. Francis from 1860–1880*, p. 19.

First Record of Covington — moved In 1868 on

ST. ELIZABETH'S HOSPITAL REGISTER. Incorpora

NAME.	RESIDENCE.	NATIVITY.	Age.	Male.	Female.	Married.	Single.	OCCUPATION.	INJURY OR DISEASE.	DISCH'GD. Month Day	Cured.	Improved.	Not imp'd.	Dead.	DATE OF DEATH. Month Day	Remaining.	
Louis Eeyer	Covington		37					Laborer									
Elizabeth Renner	Covington		21														

Louis Myer died on March 11, 1861. The cause of his death was listed as a "decay of the bones."[20] In the matter of his death, Myer was in the minority of patients at St. Elizabeth Hospital. Of the 79 patients who came to the hospital in 1861, only 13 died while in the care of the sisters. The low death rate was truly a remarkable figure, considering that most people in the 19th century went to a hospital only as a last resort.

In addition to caring for the poor and the sick who came to the hospital, the institution also filled a need it had not envisioned. Abandoned infants and young children also became part of the new hospital's mission. The first arrived in the summer of 1862 by way of Sarah Worthington Peter. She brought a newborn who was abandoned on the doorstep of St. Mary's Hospital in Cincinnati to Bishop Carrell. Carrell, in turn, promptly brought the child to the hospital. This child would be the first of many. Soon more and more children would be brought to the new hospital. The institution was taxed to the limit, but it was the only place in the region accepting infants and young children, and it soon gained a reputation as a place for unwanted children.

One story illustrates the nature of how the babies were brought to the hospital. One cold evening, a young girl came to the hospital carrying an infant and asking if the kind sisters could take the baby, her brother. The sister who answered the door informed the girl that the hospital was full and that they could not take care of any more children. The girl sighed and, since she was only a little bigger than the baby, asked the sister if she could hold the baby while she went to find her mother. The sister agreed, and the girl disappeared around the corner of the building and was never seen again.[21]

The introduction of an infant asylum to the mission of the hospital brought the first major expansion to St. Elizabeth Hospital. The nuns needed a place where crying babies and young children would not disturb the sick in the hospital. Prior to the Bishop's purchase of the St. Elizabeth hospital property in 1856, the lot on which the building was located, lot 100 in Footes addition to the city of Covington, had been subdivided. The western 25-foot portion of the 50-foot-wide lot belonged to Andrew J. Bryant and his wife, Elizabeth. The property had been purchased from Mary and Simeon Smith for the hefty sum of $4,000 in February 1861. On the half lot stood a two-story building, suitable for the orphanage, as well

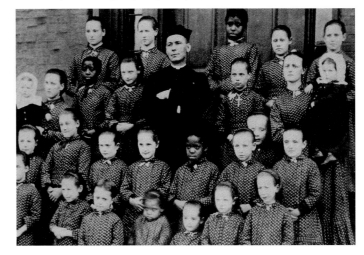

as two additional buildings on the back of the property.

The $4,000 the Bryants had paid for the property may have been more than the fledgling Diocese of Covington could readily afford, because of the continued poverty of the Catholic Church. The amount reflected almost twice the diocese's investment in St. Elizabeth Hospital. In addition, the diocese had mortgages that needed to be paid off, which greatly limited the available funds needed to purchase any more property. Indeed, in early 1862, Bishop Carrell had tendered his resignation as Bishop of Covington, due in part to the crushing debt load the diocese was under. He stated that he could no longer handle the stress. His resignation was not accepted.[22]

20 *History of St. Elizabeth Hospital, Covington, Kentucky, Under the Direction of the Sisters of the Poor of St. Francis from 1860-1880*, p. 20.

21 *History of St. Elizabeth Hospital, Covington, Kentucky, Under the Direction of the Sisters of the Poor of St. Francis from 1860-1880*, p. 33.

22 Ryan, Paul E. *History of the Diocese of Covington Kentucky*, (Covington, KY: The Diocese of Covington, 1954), p. 177.

The Sisters and the Slave

It was a cold January evening when Sister Rosa was summoned from the hospital to the home of prominent Baptist minister Thomas J. Fisher. Dressed as warmly as she could for the cold winter evening, she headed into the night. At the home she found Henrietta, an enslaved woman in her early 40s, in acute pain with what Sister Rosa knew as the last stages of "rheumatism." Rheumatism in the 1860s was a catch-all diagnosis for a number of diseases manifesting themselves in joint and body pain.

It was probably obvious to Sister Rosa that she had been called as a last resort, for it was known that Rev. Fisher had no particular love of either Catholics or slaves. Fisher was a leader in the anti-reform movement of the Baptist Church, actively arguing that baptism served no purpose in the salvation of souls and was only used after someone had consciously joined the faithful. This belief was contrary to the doctrine of the Catholic Church, where baptism is an important sacrament. Fisher was also a strong believer in predestination, the idea that human beings were so corrupt from sin that there was nothing that anyone could do to be saved and that only God's grace could save one from eternal damnation. Therefore, he believed that an act of religious devotion by those whom God had not already predestined to be saved was a waste of time and effort. This group of people included, in Fisher's opinion, those who were somehow less than fully human. To people like Fisher, this group included slaves.

Henrietta and other enslaved people, in the eyes of many slave owners like Fisher, were lesser beings who needed the yoke of slavery to help civilize them as a race. It is not clear if Fisher believed Henrietta had a soul, as many slave owners at the time did not, but at any

rate he would not allow her to pray the way she wanted to in the last days of her sickness. This fact shocked Sister Rosa and the other sisters from the hospital. They soon conspired, along with Henrietta, to have her moved to the hospital and persuaded Fisher, who reluctantly let her go.

At the hospital, Henrietta enjoyed a taste of freedom that she had never experienced before. The sisters allowed her to pray and taught her about the love of Jesus and how he

died for all mankind, so that all could be saved. Despite her sufferings, Henrietta spent the last of her days learning from the sisters and building a warm relationship with them. Toward the end of her life, she expressed a desire to be baptized into the Catholic faith. Knowing that Rev. Fisher would object to the baptism of his slave, the sisters desired to baptize the woman in secret. The action was agreed to by the priest, who performed the baptism on January 28, 1863, the day that Henrietta died.

The sisters then contacted Fisher, who had the body of Henrietta removed from the hospital and buried. He never knew of the good work the sisters at St. Elizabeth performed for Henrietta or the baptism of his slave.

History of St. Elizabeth Hospital, Covington, Kentucky, Under the Direction of the Sisters of the Poor of St. Francis from 1860–1880, handwritten text by unknown member of the order, unpublished document in private collection. p. 40.

Ledger entry for Henrietta, an enslaved woman who was secretly baptized at St. Elizabeth on January 28, 1863.

Opposite: Image of a Union fort constructed in Northern Kentucky in 1862 to defend the region against Confederate attack.

Fortunately, a number of factors had changed the cultural and economic landscape which made the purchase of the neighboring property possible. First, the start of the Civil War caused an economic crisis that forced property values in some areas of the nation to decrease. This included the area of Covington, which sat on the border between North and South. Kentucky was pro-union, but because slavery was legal in the state, there were many who supported the Southern cause. This made buying property on the south side of the Ohio River a risky investment. Secondly, Sarah Worthington King Peter, who brought the first orphan baby to St. Elizabeth Hospital, felt strongly that the care of infants and orphan children should be a function of the hospital. Fortunately, Peter had both the will and the means to make the orphanage at the hospital possible. On March 7, 1862, Bryant sold the property to Rufus King, the attorney son of Sarah Peter, for the sum of $1,400. Peter often relied upon her son, a talented and influential Cincinnati lawyer, to conduct her business affairs and to manage her charitable work. On June 27, 1862, Rufus King transferred ownership of the western half of lot 100 to Bishop Carrell for a dollar and "other considerations."[23]

The opening of the orphanage at the hospital could not have come at a better time, as the war caused not only economic hardship, but also took the lives of many fathers. Women, with little or no means of support, sought alternatives for their children and infants. In addition, in an era when medical knowledge—including pre-natal care—was limited, the infant and early childhood mortality rate was quite high, averaging more than 20 percent.[24] The Catholic Church was concerned for the bodies and souls of all infants.

The American Civil War brought additional challenges for the sisters at St. Elizabeth. In the late summer of 1862, a Confederate army marched toward Northern Kentucky and Cincinnati. Martial law was declared in the region, and the Union Army hastily erected a number of forts on the Kentucky side of the Ohio River to protect the region. These forts included Fort Wright, Fort Mitchell and a number of artillery emplacements. The late summer heat made the task difficult, and a number

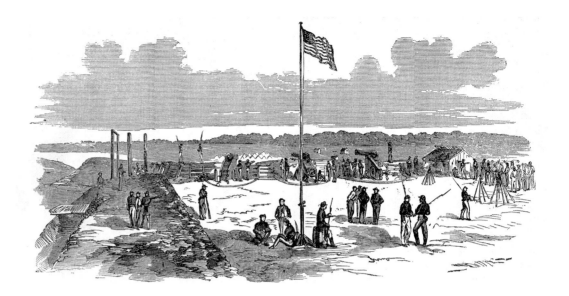

of soldiers suffered from dysentery and heat exhaustion. Twenty-seven sick soldiers were sent to St. Elizabeth Hospital to recover.

The soldiers brought other challenges to the young sisters at the hospital. Being young men, they had large appetites for food and drink. The sisters who supported the hospital by begging door-to-door found the additional burden difficult. Sister Rosa was most often sent out to beg for food for the hospital. As one of her fellow sisters said, "What she did not bring home we did not eat."[25] Fortunately, Bishop Carrell always saw to it that the soldiers at the hospital had enough to eat by bringing ex-

tra food to the hospital whenever possible. At one point, Sister Agnus and Sister Ann were sent out to beg for "spirituous liquors" for the soldiers. They were unsuccessful in their mission and returned to the hospital empty-handed.[26]

The first few years of St. Elizabeth Hospital's existence were difficult. There were constant shortages of money, food and fuel, as well as persistent fears of fire and Confederate invasion. The one thing that the sisters had in abundance were patients. In the first year, the sisters had 107 people at various times in the hospital, not including infants and children in the hospital's orphanage. During the years 1862 and 1863

23 Deed Book 3, pp. 478–480, Andrew Bryant to Rufus King and Rufus King to George Carrell, Kenton County Courthouse, Covington, Kentucky.

24 Steckel, Richard H. "The Health and Mortality of Women and Children, 1850–1860," *The Journal of Economic History*, vol. 48, no. 2 (June 1988), p. 334.

25 *History of St. Elizabeth Hospital, Covington, Kentucky, Under the Direction of the Sisters of the Poor of St. Francis from 1860–1880*, p. 50.

26 *History of St. Elizabeth Hospital, Covington, Kentucky, Under the Direction of the Sisters of the Poor of St. Francis from 1860–1880*, pp. 38–39.

the hospital served 76 and 78 patients a year, respectively, a remarkable feat considering that the hospital had officially only 10 patient beds. During these early years, the death rate averaged between 15 and 18 annually, indicating that despite the overwhelming hardships and the lack of certain advantages of other institutions, the small hospital was about average for the nation.

The Civil War and the continued growth of the cities of Northern Kentucky taxed the small hospital nearly to the breaking point. During the hospital's first years of existence, the main source of support for St. Elizabeth was a variety of street fairs, concerts and outright begging by the sisters. As time when on, problems arose making the task of raising money more difficult. The sisters at the hospital developed a dislike for street fairs because of the potential for corruption at the events.[27] Begging also became problematic as criminals went door-to-door soliciting funds in the name of the hospital. The problem became so acute that St. Elizabeth Hospital had to run an ad in the *Covington Journal* saying that only persons carrying official letters from the Mother Superior were allowed to solicit funds in the name of the hospital.[28]

The criminal attempts to obtain a portion of the money collected by the sisters

---

27 *History of St. Elizabeth Hospital, Covington, Kentucky, Under the Direction of the Sisters of the Poor of St. Francis from 1860–1880,* p. 17.

28 *Covington Journal,* September 26, 1868.

Medical Advice, 1800s Style

Getting Rid of Bedbugs

It is not known what the sisters at the first St. Elizabeth Hospital used to get rid of the bedbugs, but the Workwoman's Guide published in 1838 offered the advice below. Please do not try this at home since quicksilver (mercury) is highly toxic to humans as well as to insects.

Mix some quicksilver (mercury) in a mortar with the white of an egg, till the quicksilver is all mixed, and there are no bubbles; then beat up the white of another egg, and put it to the mixture in the mortar, until it becomes a fine ointment.

Anoint the bedstead all over in every crack with a brush and put it also about the cord lacing and headboard. When repeated for two or three following days, the cure will be effectual and bedstead uninjured.

Coffee

Strong black coffee, the beans being little roasted and drunk as hot as possible, is indispensible for a large number of poisons, especially from those that cause drowsiness, intoxication, loss of consciousness or mental derangement or delirium.

An Epitome of the Homeopathic Healing Art, Containing the New Discoveries and Improvements to the Present Time; Designed for the use of Families and Travelers and as a Pocket Companion for the Physician, 11th Edition, by B. L. Hill, M.D. (Professor of General, Special and Surgical Anatomy, late Professor of Surgery, Obstetrics, and Diseases of Women and Children, in the W.H. College, Author of the "Homeopathic Practice of Surgery" & c., & c., 1864. P. 131.

---

and supporters of the hospital were a testimony to how popular and important the hospital had become. Not only were the beds at the hospital constantly full, but often the sisters were called upon to help those who could not make it to the hospital or to visit sick persons at home when the hospital was at capacity. In one such case, Sister Rosa was called to the former Baptist seminary on 11th Street, which had been converted to a hospital for sick or injured soldiers of the Civil War. In 1863 a smallpox epidemic swept Cincinnati and Northern Kentucky, affecting many soldiers.

Nurses at the military hospital, including the head nurse, contracted the highly contagious disease while treating the patients in their care. As a result, word was sent to St. Elizabeth for all the help that they could spare, which amounted to Sister Antonia. The good sister was impressed with the 100-bed facility and commented how wonderful it would be as a community hospital. Little did she know she was looking into the future of St. Elizabeth Hospital.

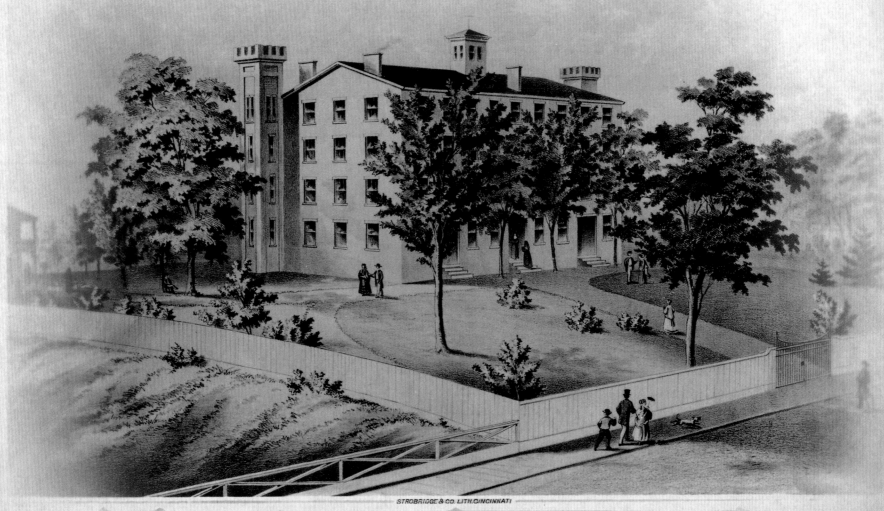

STROBRIDGE & CO. LITH. CINCINNATI

Rec.d of M_____ Dollars_____ for the Benefit of the

ST. ELIZABETH HOSPITAL,
COVINGTON, KY.

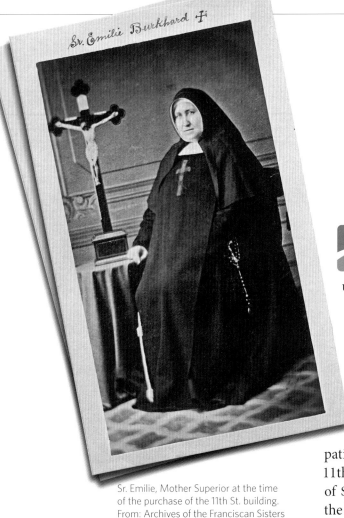

Sr. Emilie Burkhard ✝

Sr. Emilie, Mother Superior at the time of the purchase of the 11th St. building. From: Archives of the Franciscan Sisters of the Poor, Hartwell (Cincinnati), Ohio.

Opposite: Western Baptist Theological Institute, 11th St., Covington, became the second location of St. Elizabeth Hospital. From: Richard H. Collins, *History of Kentucky* (1874), volume 2.

Previous page: Lithograph of St. Elizabeth Hospital on 11th St. in Covington. The sisters added small, castle-like additions that contained 4-story privies. From: Kenton County Public Library, Covington.

According to the *Covington Journal* in 1868, a few years earlier the managers of St. Elizabeth Hospital had faced a very difficult choice: they could continue as they were in the Seventh Street building—overcrowded and under-supported—eventually collapsing under the sheer weight of the community's needs, or they could move to better quarters and grow with the city. The sisters and their supporters kept their eyes open for any type of building or land to build on that would suit their needs. Fortunately for St. Elizabeth Hospital, the sisters who managed it and the people of Northern Kentucky, opportunity came knocking.

One day, Sister Rosa returned from her rounds of sick patients in their homes with some exciting news: a fine building on 11th Street could be purchased for the incredibly reasonable price of $15,000. Mother Superior Emilie requested to be taken to see the building immediately.[1] Ironically, it was the same building that Sister Rosa had seen before when helping out in the smallpox epidemic during the Civil War. The structure was the former Baptist Seminary building that had been used as a hospital by the Union Army during the war.

What Sister Emilie saw pleased her. The large building, built of substantial brick, was four stories tall and had plenty of room on

1 *History of St. Elizabeth Hospital, Covington, Kentucky, Under the Direction of the Sisters of the Poor of St. Francis from 1860–1880*, handwritten text by unknown member of the order, unpublished document in private collection, p. 87.

the grounds. She also saw that the building had been allowed to sit vacant for a number of years. The fence surrounding the building had been knocked over and wild pigs were now living on the grounds. Despite this, she judged the building to be perfect for a hospital and immediately took steps to view the interior of the structure.[2]

The sisters felt that exploring the possibility of obtaining the building for a new hospital needed to be done in secret. This may have been for two reasons. First, show-

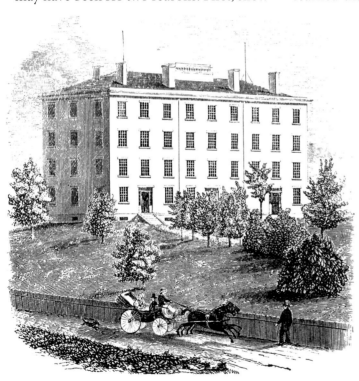

ing interest in the building might drive up the price. Also, the sisters may have feared that anti-Catholic sentiment, still strong in the city, would prevent them from purchasing the property. In order to avoid these possibilities, Sister Emilie solicited the help of Henrietta Scott Cleveland, who pretended to be interested in renting the building as a cover for the sisters' investigation of the property.[3]

After visiting the site again, the sisters learned that the manager for the property was a Mr. Kopper, who resided in Covington, and that John B. Temple in Frankfort was the true administrator of the property. Temple was the executor for the estate of Thomas D. Carneal of Frankfort. They also learned that the true selling price for the building was not the $15,000 that Sister Rosa had reported but actually $50,000. Temple set his terms that the building would be paid for within three years at an interest rate of 6 percent on the unpaid balance. The sisters would need to pay $12,500 up front to close the deal, with the rest being paid in yearly

installments over the next three years. In total, the sisters would pay $54,000 for the property. This figure did not include what expenses it would take to convert the building into a first-class hospital.

When the sisters reported their findings to the leaders of the Diocese of Covington, they must have thought the good sisters had lost their minds. How could the sisters of St. Elizabeth Hospital and their supporters come up with more than $50,000 when they were barely able to support the small hospital they already managed? Naysayers took their complaints to the Bishop, stating that "the sisters don't know anything," and that they were getting in way over their heads.[4] The Bishop heard the complaints and dismissed them. Perhaps his witnessing of what the sisters had already done convinced him that they could do anything that they set their minds to. With little more than their zeal for the project and the belief that God was on their side, the sisters moved forward on the purchase of the property on 11th Street.

The sisters needed to start raising money as quickly as they could, including finding four wealthy Catholic supporters who were willing to back the loans the sisters would obtain to get the funds needed for purchase. After much persuading and help from Rev. Conrad Rother, four individu-

---

2 *History of St. Elizabeth Hospital, Covington, Kentucky, Under the Direction of the Sisters of the Poor of St. Francis from 1860–1880,* pp. 87–88.

3 *History of St. Elizabeth Hospital, Covington, Kentucky,* p. 87.

4 *History of St. Elizabeth Hospital, Covington, Kentucky, Under the Direction of the Sisters of the Poor of St. Francis from 1860–1880,* p. 90.

als stepped forward to support the new hospital project. Willing to put up their personal fortunes as collateral for the sisters' loans were Henry Drexelius, a wealthy tailor; Johann Schmitt, a famous Catholic artist; Henry Meyer, a bank manager; and Clement Hellenbusch, a jeweler and silversmith.[5]

However, another challenge faced the supporters of the 11th Street hospital project. In the eyes of the state of Kentucky, the Sisters of the Poor of St. Francis did not legally exist because their order had not officially incorporated as an organization in the United States or in the state of Kentucky. As such, the sisters could not enter into legal contracts, purchase property or even solicit funds.

In 1868 the law required four individuals willing to sign as incorporators in order to create a corporation within the state of Kentucky. The four nuns who signed the legal documents required by the state were Sister Emilie Bruchard, Sister Paula Nellessen, Sister Placida V. Alst and Sister Antonia Goeb. The name of the corporation would be the Sisters of the Poor of St. Francis, Covington.[6] The corporation would follow a perpetual succession and have the authority to "take and to hold such property, real and personal, goods and chattels not exceeding 200,000 dollars." The document was signed by the speaker of the Kentucky House of Representatives, the speaker of the Senate, the governor and the secretary of state. In March 1868, the Sisters of the Poor of St. Francis, Covington became a Kentucky corporation.

While the process of becoming a Kentucky corporation was going on, the sisters were far from idle. The building needed to be secured for the sisters and money needed to be raised. Pledges of support came in. Ministers, both Catholic and Protestant, preached to their congregations about the benefits of supporting the hospital. The city of Covington pledged $5,000 on September 21, 1868, toward the new hospital, and benefit concerts were organized by Henrietta Cleveland at the Odd Fellows Hall. The price of admission to the concert was 50 cents, a hefty amount for the average citizen.[7]

Rev. Rother served as agent for the sisters and entered a contract to purchase the building from the Carneal estate. In a deed dated November 11, 1867, Rother, on behalf of the sisters, pledged to pay off the mortgage in an agreed upon timetable, thus placing a lien on the property.[8] He also paid the first $12,500, representing the first of four payments needed to purchase the property. Because the sisters could not hold the property as an institution, but only as individuals, Father Rother became the official owner of the building. Had one of the sisters agreed to be the owner of the property while the order was incorporated, it

Johann Schmitt (1825-1898), a famous artist of Covington, was among the four men who guaranteed the mortgage for the purchase of the 11th St. hospital. He also painted the murals for the chapel there. From: Sharon Cahill.

Opposite: St. Elizabeth Hospital, 11th St., Covington, circa 1909. From: Paul A. Tenkotte, Ph.D.

5 1870 United States Census for the City of Covington, Ward 4.

6 Original incorporation document, "The Sisters of the Poor of St. Francis, Covington" located in the archives of the Sisters of St. Francis of the Poor archive at Hartwell, Cincinnati, Ohio.

7 *Covington Journal*, October 10, 1868.

8 Kenton County Deed Book 16, pp. 482–483, Covington Courthouse.

would have been a violation of the sisters' vow of poverty. Rother would continue to own the building until the sisters officially became a legal corporation. He transferred ownership to them on May 22, 1868, the day before the building was officially dedicated.[9] In exchange for this kindness, the sisters pledged to take care of him for the rest of his life, either by being given a permanent home in the new hospital or any other facility owned by the sisters as long as he so desired.[10]

But things were not going as well as the sisters would have wanted. There was considerable opposition to the idea of a new hospital. Part of the opposition may have been the age-old fear that a hospital would bring diseases into the community. However, the principal opposition seemed to have been based on anti-Catholic sentiment, still very much alive in the city at the time.

On September 23, 1868, William Ernst (1813–1895) and others filed a lawsuit against the city of Covington in order to stop the city from paying its pledge of $5,000 to the new St. Elizabeth Hospital.[11] Ernst's official complaint was that if the city were to pay the $5,000 to a Catholic

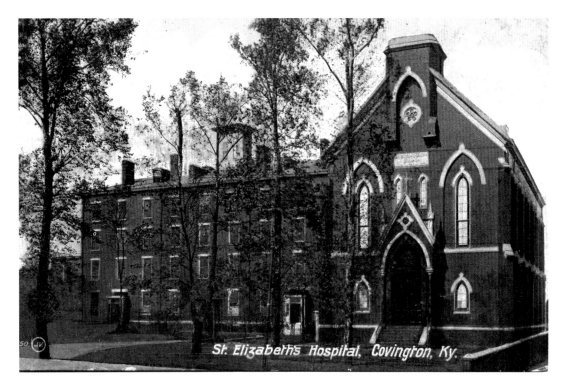

St. Elizabeth's Hospital, Covington, Ky.

hospital, it would be the same as paying the money to the Catholic Church, which would set a dangerous precedent. Soon, Ernst and his supporters argued, the city would be besieged by Methodists, Baptists and other various denominations looking for a handout. This act also would threaten the separation of church and state.

At the time of the lawsuit, Ernst was the president of the Covington branch of the Northern Bank of Kentucky, a position he held until 1888. Later, he served as president of the Covington City Council, president of the Covington and Lexington Turnpike Company and treasurer of the

Kentucky Central Railroad. He was one of the founders of the First Presbyterian Church of Covington, where he served as an elder for 50 years and sang in the choir. It was said he had a beautiful voice. One of his sons, Richard Pretlow Ernst, became a United States senator from Kentucky.[12]

Almost as soon as Ernst filed his lawsuit against the city, arguments for and against the donation to the hospital appeared in local newspapers. Accusations flew in both directions. One Covington city councilman

9 Kenton County Deed Book 17, pp. 564-566, Covington Courthouse.

10 *History of St. Elizabeth Hospital, Covington, Kentucky, Under the Direction of the Sisters of the Poor of St. Francis from 1860-1880*, handwritten text by unknown member of the order, unpublished document in private collection, p. 124

11 Records of the Kenton County Circuit Court, September term, 1868, pp. 127, 200, 209, 239, 261.

12 Tenkotte, Paul A. and James C. Claypool, *Encyclopedia of Northern Kentucky*, (Lexington: The University Press of Kentucky, 2009), pp. 311-312.

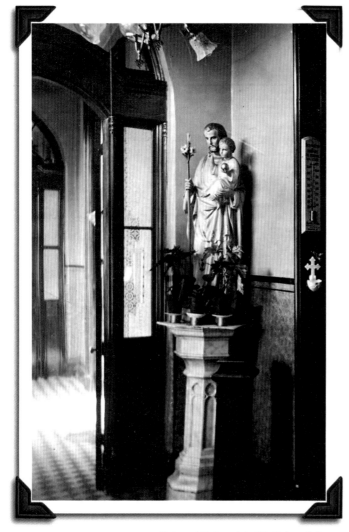

Statue of St. Joseph in 11th St. hospital.
From: St. Elizabeth Healthcare.

Right: Sisters Eusebia *(left)* and Radigundis *(right)* served many years at St. Elizabeth Hospital. Sr. Radigundis assisted in the move of the hospital from 11th St. to 20th St. Date of photo is unknown as well as whether Sr. Eusebia served at 11th St. From: St. Elizabeth Healthcare.

defended the hospital, saying that although the institution was managed by Catholic sisters, it served the entire community regardless of race, religious affiliation or ability to pay. The writer went on to ask if it was not the obligation of all the followers of Christ to care for their fellow human beings. In a final statement the councilman's letter made a comment that was perhaps aimed at William Ernst. The writer said he would not object to supporting a project that had the goal of universal charity and benevolence even if the source was Presbyterian, Baptist or something else.[13] Sadly, in the same newspaper where this argument was unfolding, it was reported that Bishop George Aloysius Carrell had died at his residence. St. Elizabeth Hospital had lost one of its truest and dearest friends.

On October 3, 1868, the *Covington Journal* reported several important events related to St. Elizabeth Hospital. The major story was the funeral of Bishop Carrell, the description of which went on for several columns. There was also a copy of a letter written to the City Council by Sister Emilie, Mother Superior of St. Elizabeth Hospital, accepting the city's pledge of $5,000 in exchange for the exclusive use of five beds in the new hospital for patients sent there by the city of Covington. These beds, presumably, would be

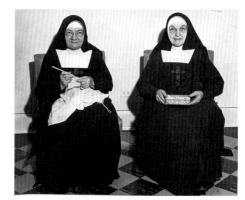

set aside for poor people who were receiving aid from the city. One more item in the paper reported on a resolution passed by the City Council to affirm the donation to the hospital and to order the city attorney to oppose the lawsuit put forth by William Ernst and others. The resolution further authorized the city attorney to employ attorney John G. Carlisle to assist in fighting the suit if needed.

---

13 *Covington Journal*, September 26, 1868.

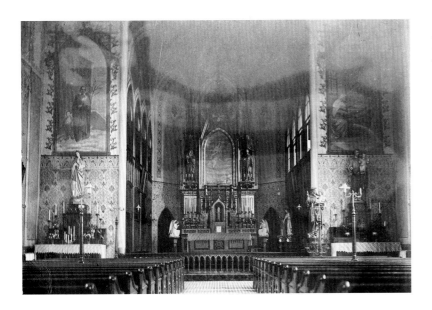

The tactic used by Ernst and his followers was to tie up the donation to St. Elizabeth by gaining one continuance after another in court. The first was to allow the plaintiff, Ernst, to complete the needed paperwork on the suit; another was granted to allow the filing of further amendments and affidavits. Perhaps it was the hope of William Ernst and his followers to draw out the process long enough for it to become an embarrassment to Sister Emilie and the supporters of St. Elizabeth Hospital. Whether or not this was the purpose of their actions is unknown, but it was the result. On December 24, 1868, Sister Emilie informed the Kenton County Circuit Court that she and St. Elizabeth Hospital would relinquish all claims to the city's donation, thus ending the lawsuit.

With the conclusion of the lawsuit, the sisters' effort to win over many of the citizens continued, as did conflicts. However, the sisters' gentle and persistent drive in the face of adversity gained many supporters. In at least one case, the sisters gained a supporter by what can only be referred to as an ironic twist of fate, clearly showing that God has a sense of humor. According to a newspaper account, one day, one of the sisters was out looking for food donations for the hospital and saw a man digging potatoes out of his garden. Hoping to gain a gift of some of the potatoes for the patients at St. Elizabeth, she approached the man. The man, upon hearing her request, abruptly told her that he had "nothing to give to Catholics!" Before leaving, the sister informed the man that St. Elizabeth Hospital was open to people of all faiths or no faith at all. Anyone who was in need was welcome at the hospital. Not long after the conversation with the sister, the man was seriously wounded in a hunting accident when his gun went off unexpectedly. Because his family was not at home, the man's friends carried him to St. Elizabeth Hospital." Upon his regaining consciousness, the first face he saw was the sister who had asked him for the potatoes. According to

BASEBALL!

The Glorys and the White Swans will cross bats at the Willow Run, Sunday afternoon.

The Ludlows and the Kentons of this city will play a match game for a stake on the grounds of the Kentons on Sunday afternoon. Game will be called at 2:30 sharp.

Yesterday at St. Louis, Cincinnati 4, St. Louis 1; at Chicago, Chicago 7, Troy 1; at Cleveland, Providence 2, Cleveland 0; at Detroit, Boston 10, Detroit 3; at Buffalo, Buffalo 10, Worcester 1; at Baltimore, Allegheny 7, Baltimore 5.

The "laugh-ats" of this city have reorganized, and are open for any challenge from nines who may want to cross bats with them. The names are, Captain, William Kleist; Secretary, A. Mahone. The nine—Ed. Bristler, c; A. Mahone, p; A. Cummins, s. s; W. Hackathorn, 1st b; J. Shoup, 2nd b; C. Crimmons, 3rd b; L. Applegate, l.f; W. Kieith, c.f; J. Sommer, r.f.

Daily Commonwealth, September 8, 1882

Left: Interior of chapel, hospital on 11th St. Note murals by Johann Schmitt. From: St. Elizabeth Healthcare.

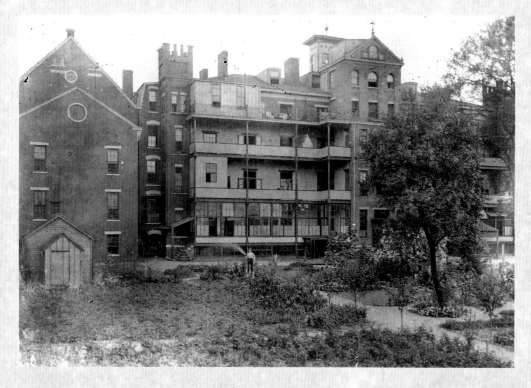

Rear of St. Elizabeth Hospital on 11th St., including the gardens, a portion of the orchard and the small building at the left behind the chapel (dead house). From: Kenton County Public Library, Covington.

Opposite: 1896 Sanborn Insurance Map showing St. Elizabeth Hospital on 11th St. Note small building marked "Dead House" behind the chapel. From: Kenton County Public Library, Covington.

the account, "He is now a liberal contributor and fast friend of the hospital."[14]

In addition to the $54,000 needed to purchase the building, the sisters spent $20,000 on physical improvements.[15] These improvements included a new roof, a heating system, a water pipe system designed to allow water to be accessible in all parts of the building, and two towers in the corners of the structure to serve as four-story outhouses. The "towers", as they were referred to by the sisters, were built so that sick patients and nurses carrying bedpans would not have to

leave the floor they were on to make use of the restroom. Ironically, although the building was "piped" for running water, the city at the time had no sewer or water system. The hospital needed to wait for the city to catch up with the modern conveniences of St. Elizabeth Hospital.[16]

The new St. Elizabeth Hospital sat on a large lot located on the north side of 11th Street between the tracks of the Covington and Lexington Railroad and Washington Street. The building contained 54 large rooms and had a capacity of approximately 100 beds. The nuns' rooms and kitchen were located on the west side of the building. Immediately to the right as one entered the building was a small chapel that served until a larger chapel was built on the east side of the grounds. Each floor had a main hallway that ran the width of the building, and each hallway contained a staircase. On the fourth floor, a small staircase led to a small tower or cupola on the roof, which contained a small bell and cross. One of the major inconveniences of the building's interior was that there was a central hall running the length of the building on each floor. Nurses and nuns working to aid patients had to walk through other patient rooms to get to where they were going.[17]

The grounds of the hospital were one of the major attractions of the building. The large open land allowed for a kitchen garden and an orchard.

14 *The Ticket*, October 2, 1877.

15 *Covington Journal*, May 23, 1868.

16 *History of St. Elizabeth Hospital, Covington, Kentucky, Under the Direction of the Sisters of the Poor of St. Francis from 1860–1880*, p. 121.

17 *History of St. Elizabeth Hospital, Covington, Kentucky, Under the Direction of the Sisters of the Poor of St. Francis from 1860–1880*, pp. 127-128.

The sisters often kept a large iron pot cooking over an open fire in the yard. In the pot went anything and everything that the sisters could collect in the way of food. With the large pot on hand and always cooking, it provided a constant supply of stew for the patients when other sources of food ran short.

Maps of the city between 1877 and 1900 clearly show the building and grounds of the hospital. In addition to the hospital and the chapel, there were a number of other buildings on the site. One structure, built on the back of the lot on 10th Street, was labeled a carpentry shop but was probably originally built as a stable. There were also buildings listed as a greenhouse, a guest house, a children's house, a chicken coop and two "dead houses."[18] The reference to

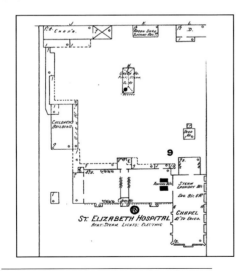

Conversion by Fear

Sister Beatrix tells the story of a tough railroad worker who repented due to a fright. The worker was brought to St. Elizabeth because of an injury. He told the nuns that he was a Catholic but was not interested in taking the sacraments or expressing any nature of religious belief. When asked if he wanted to participate in worship he told the nuns that he would "wait until I get well again, then I will go to church." One night when Sister Beatrix was in charge of the hospital she made her rounds and then went to her office. After working a while, she was disturbed by a rapping on the window by the night attendant. She waved him off, but he became more agitated, gaining her attention. He reported that a black woman with a lantern had gotten into the men's side of the hospital and was scaring everybody. Especially scared was the tough railroader who had no time for religion.

Upon her arrival in the ward, Sister Beatrix found the woman chasing the railroader from room to room and the man screaming with fear, much to the delight of his fellow ward-mates.

It seemed that the poor woman, delirious with fever, had somehow gotten hold of a lantern and walked into the men's ward. Out of pure chance she approached the sleeping railroader, and with her face close to the lantern, touched the warm lantern to the man's face. This immediately woke him up. The first thing he saw was the woman's face illuminated by the red glow of the lantern. Remembering the heat of the lantern, the only conclusion the man could come to was the devil had come to claim his soul. He jumped from the bed with the woman in hot pursuit. He ran to and fro begging for forgiveness, pleading for the Lord to have mercy on his sinful soul. Sister Beatrix and the attendant helped return the girl to the women's ward and the repentant railroad worker to his bed. His ward-mates, who had recognized the woman as a female patient of the hospital, teased the railroad worker about his run-in with the "devil."

True to his word however, the man repented his sins, went to confession and turned his life around.

History of St. Elizabeth Hospital, Covington, Kentucky, Under the Direction of the Sisters of the Poor of St. Francis from 1860–1880, handwritten text by unknown member of the order, unpublished document in private collection, p. 201.

the "dead houses" may reflect a series of sensational events that took place in the Cincinnati area involving body snatching.

On May 28, 1878, future President Benjamin Harrison attended the funeral of his father, John Scott Harrison, son of former President William Henry Harrison. While at the funeral he learned that the body of another relative, a young man who died just a few days before, was missing from his grave. Fearing the body had been stolen for medical study by the Medical College

of Ohio, a day or two later members of the Harrison family sought legal warrants to allow them to seek the body. An early morning raid of the college did not reveal the young man's body, but the searches found dozens of bodies, including the newly arrived body of John Scott Harrison hanging by his neck in a delivery chute.[19]

The resulting investigation and trial

revealed that the Cincinnati and Northern Kentucky area was a center for body snatching. The earthly remains of thousands of dead Ohio Valley residents were being shipped all over the Midwest to medical schools willing to pay the price and look the other way. One of the biggest clients for illegally stolen bodies was the University of Michigan.

The sensational trial caused a virtual panic among the citizenry. Armed guards were hired to protect new graves, cemeteries built special vaults to keep bodies until they had decayed to the point to not be any use to thieves, and enterprising inventors developed devices that would explode if graves were tampered with. Hospitals, like St. Elizabeth in Covington, had to take extra precautions to prevent the stealing of bodies. To the sisters in the leadership of the hospital, it was both a moral and a religious issue. This may explain the two buildings marked "dead houses" on the insurance maps, 1886–1894, on the hospital grounds.

The hospital was dedicated on May 24, 1868. Of the many religious and civic dignitaries on hand, probably the most important was Sister Frances Schervier, who traveled to America just for the dedication. Her visit greatly lifted the spirits of the sisters at the hospital, and unlike her previous journey in 1863 when she visited only for a short time at the Seventh Street hospital, she stayed at the new hospital several weeks. While there, she visited patients, convers-

ing with many in her native German language. She took particular interest in the many children and infants in the hospital. She paid particular attention to a dying

For the Sake of the Children

The *Covington Journal* on October 3, 1868, reported that physiologists have complained to the New York school system that they are overworking the brains of children, which will lead to idiocy and death. Less algebra and more romp is advised.

black infant whom she sponsored in baptism and named Francis. Mother Schervier stayed with the child many days without rest, giving the child comfort until the baby passed on.

Schervier took particular pleasure in the fact that the hospital had once been a Baptist seminary. During the dedication, when it was mentioned that the building had once belonged to the Baptists, she reportedly leaned over to sister Emilie sitting next to her and said with obvious glee, "Oh yes, dear St. Elizabeth has triumphed over the Baptists."[20] Over the next several days Mother Schervier never failed to get a chuckle whenever she saw the cornerstone

of the new hospital that read, "Baptist College, 1840."[21]

Despite the cheery and inspirational visit of Mother Schervier and the success of the dedication, the next few years of the hospital were anything but easy. Each time there was another payment due or an internal improvement that needed to be paid for, Sister Emilie struggled to find the money to keep the operation going. Miracle upon miracle seemed to happen just as all hope was about lost. One time, a poor old widower by the name of Jacob Winkler, who was staying full-time at the hospital, approached the good sister and handed her $2,057.50 for no reason, telling her that it was a gift. Ironically, that very day Sister Emilie had been trying to find a way to ask the Diocese of Covington for a loan of $2,000 in order to pay a bill that was due that evening.[22] Events like this happened time and time again, not only enabling the hospital to meet its financial obligations but also lifting the spirits of the nuns and their supporters. The nuns working at the hospital during these tough early years included: Sisters Emilie, Placida, Rosa, Angela, Sabina I, Martina I, Thecla, Blandina, Gutta I, Beata I, Bonaventure I, Aegidia, Ursula I, and Hyacinth.[23]

20 *History of St. Elizabeth Hospital, Covington, Kentucky, Under the Direction of the Sisters of the Poor of St. Francis from 1860–1880*, p. 125.

21 *History of St. Elizabeth Hospital*, Covington, Kentucky, p. 135.

22 *History of St. Elizabeth Hospital*, Covington, Kentucky, p. 139.

23 *History of St. Elizabeth Hospital*, Covington, Kentucky, pp. 119 and 144.

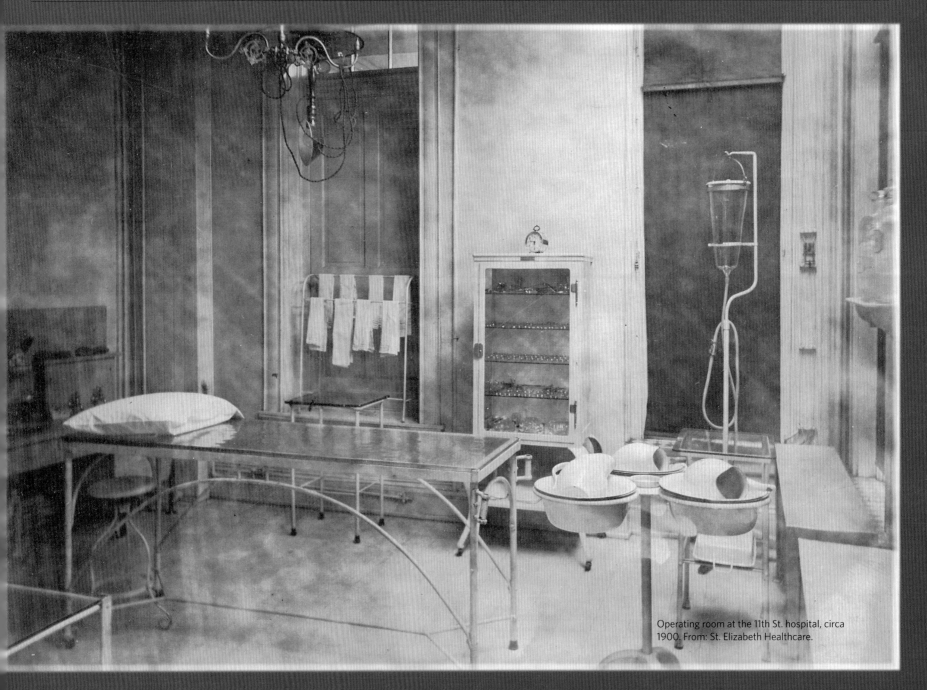

Operating room at the 11th St. hospital, circa 1900. From: St. Elizabeth Healthcare.

Probably the greatest miracle to transpire during the first years of the 11th Street hospital was the change in attitude of the people of Covington. The hospital always

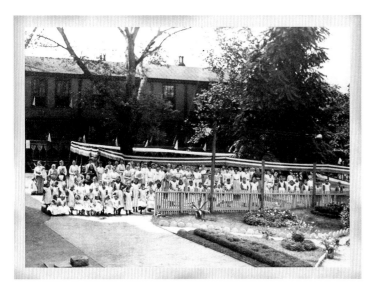

1903 picnic for the benefit of the foundlings of St. Elizabeth Hospital. From: St. Elizabeth Healthcare.

had its supporters, but there were many who were hostile to the idea of a hospital, especially one managed by Catholics. Over time, whether it was by the gentle example of the sisters or the changing nature of the community, St. Elizabeth Hospital changed from being thought of as just a feature of the city to being a part of the city. In other words, St. Elizabeth became part of the fabric of Northern Kentucky, not just a building in the city. The result was that people began to think of St. Elizabeth as their hospital, not just a hospital in their midst. This

made raising funds and getting the attention of city leaders much easier.

In February 1870, Sister Emilie began making plans for a chapel addition to the hospital. The chapel inside the hospital was much too small and needed to be replaced. The St. Vincent Society, founded a few years earlier to support the hospital, took a leadership role in raising the needed funds. Work on the chapel began in June of 1870 but was temporarily halted because of complaints by local priests. The priests were concerned that the chapel would be so grand that many worshippers would attend there rather than their home churches.[24] The priests approached the Bishop, who ordered a stop to the work until the plans for the chapel could be toned down, making it a less grand structure. One of the changes included the elimination of a bell tower from the original design. Reluctantly, the sisters at St. Elizabeth Hospital accepted the change and the chapel was completed in early 1871.

At the end of December 1869, the hospital records reported 22 patients in the building, twice the capacity of the Seventh Street building. In all, the nuns had 129

patients admitted during the year, not including patients whom they visited in their homes or in the community "pest" house, where poor people with communicable diseases were sent by county officials.[25] Ten years later when St. Elizabeth issued its first annual report, it stated that the hospital admitted 386 patients, a 300 percent increase in just 10 years. Of that number only 26 had died, a remarkable feat given the seriousness of the patients sent to the hospital.[26] The report also listed five doctors on staff. They were: Dr. Charles Kearns, surgeon and chief of staff; Dr. W.W. Dawson, consulting surgeon; Dr. E. Williams, oculist; Dr. D. F. H. Noonan, general physician; and Dr. A. Knollmann, general physician.

The coming of the 20th century brought remarkable changes to the entire medical profession as well as St. Elizabeth Hospital. The hospital that would "stand for the centuries" barely made it for a mere 42 years. The requirements of a modern hospital—science laboratories, surgical rooms, children's wards and a professionally trained staff—taxed the 11th Street hospital to the breaking point. In addition, the hospital's location next to a busy railroad line brought noise and smoke into the building from passing steam trains. By 1909, St. Elizabeth Hospital, that is to say "Covington's hospital," needed a new home.

24 *History of St. Elizabeth Hospital*, Covington, Kentucky, p. 195.

25 *History of St. Elizabeth Hospital*, Covington, Kentucky, p. 191.
26 *History of St. Elizabeth Hospital*, Covington, Kentucky, p. 313.

Chapter 4

The 20th Street Hospital

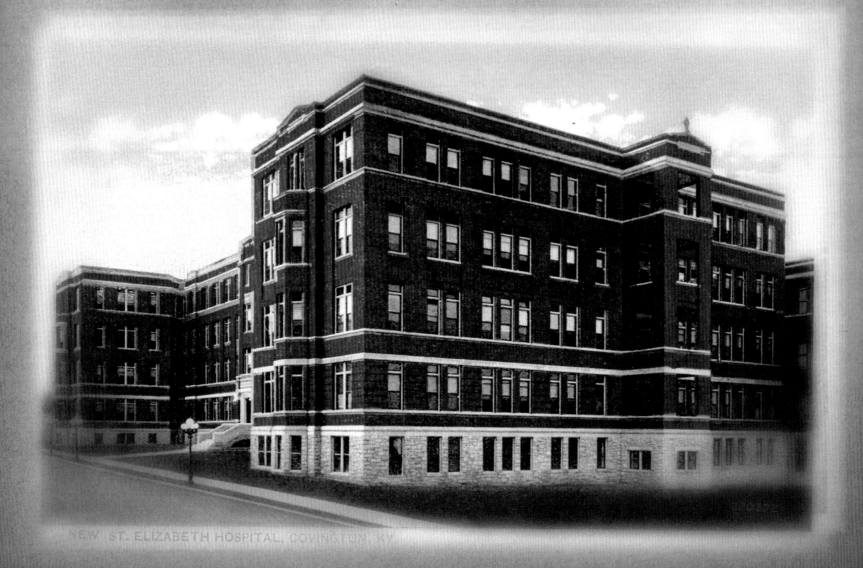

NEW ST. ELIZABETH HOSPITAL, COVINGTON, KY

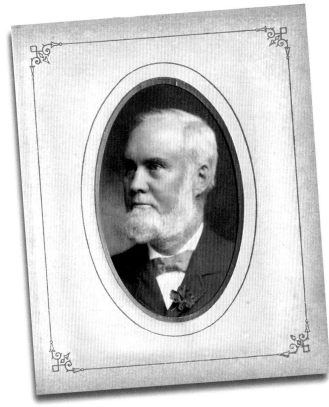

Samuel Hannaford, founder of the firm that designed the third St. Elizabeth Hospital, located between 20th and 21st Streets. From: Notable Men of Cincinnati (1903).

Opposite: St. Elizabeth Nursing School, students enrolled in 1915. From: St. Elizabeth Healthcare.

Previous page: The third location of St. Elizabeth Hospital, Covington, circa 1915. This view shows the 21st Street entrance, which functioned as the main entrance for many years. From: Paul A. Tenkotte, Ph.D.

In 1909 land was acquired in the Covington block bounded by 20th Street on the north, 21st Street on the south, Eastern Avenue on the east, and Denver Street on the west for the new St. Elizabeth Hospital. As before, with the Seventh and 11th Street buildings, the sisters leading the hospital put their faith in God and took a large and unsecured leap forward. The hospital would be a magnificent structure, eventually taking up the entire block, designed by noted architects Samuel Hannaford and Sons. Hannaford and Sons designed a number of important Cincinnati area buildings including Cincinnati City Hall, Our Lady of Providence Academy in Newport, Salem United Methodist Church in Newport, St. Bernard Catholic Church in Dayton and the Altamont Hotel in Fort Thomas.[1] Ground was broken for the new hospital in June 1911, but work was halted soon after the foundation was laid due to lack of funding.

In decades past, the Sisters of the Poor would wait until more money came in before work could continue, but things were different now. St. Elizabeth Hospital was not the struggling medical anomaly it had once been; it was now a critical part of a growing

---

1 Tenkotte, Paul and James C. Claypool, editors *"Hannaford, Samuel and Sons," The Encyclopedia of Northern Kentucky*, pp. 430–431.

and vibrant community. Covington was not going to sit back and wait for small miracles to happen in order see the hospital completed. Something had to be done and done quickly.

Frank Tracy, a prominent lawyer, judge and politician, organized what can only be described as a "whirlwind" fundraising campaign.[2] Tracy and his team of volunteers organized a fund drive that left no good idea behind. They sent solicitors door to door, held a bazaar at the site of the new hospital and ran popularity contests with prizes that ranged from diamond rings to live goats.[3] The entire city seemed to be at a fever pitch to raise money. In a little over a week, the effort had exceeded its goal of $100,000 and work again resumed on the new St. Elizabeth Hospital.

The completed hospital was dedicated on August 1, 1914, and opened to the public for inspection the next day.[4] The visiting crowd was estimated at 15,000, approximately one-fourth of the entire population of the city of Covington at the time. St. Elizabeth was certainly their hospital and they were going to enjoy it. Reports at the time indicated that people lingered in the new four-story hospital admiring

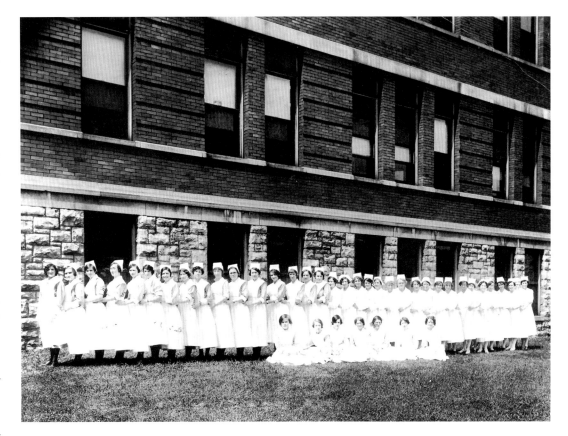

the rooms, the spacious corridors and the state-of-the-art X-ray room. Most importantly, the new hospital offered a 340-bed capacity, more than three times that of the old St. Elizabeth.

The physical structure of St. Elizabeth was not the only new thing. With the coming of the 20th century, new ideas were taking hold in the medical profession. The practice of healthcare was as much a product of science and education as it was caring. Medical schools demanded more of

their students and new areas of medical specialty were developing at an accelerated rate. Likewise, other aspects of medicine were becoming more professional. In 1915 the staff doctors at St. Elizabeth lobbied Sister Michaela Schappert to open a nursing school for the training of professional nurses. Professional nurses challenged the long-held notion that nursing was little more than the caring and nurturing for the sick, an occupation that was derived out of a woman's natural instinct. The idea that

---

2 *St. Elizabeth Medical Center: 125 Years of Caring, 1861–1986*, pp. 11–12.

3 *St. Elizabeth Medical Center: 125 Years of Caring, 1861–1986*, p. 12

4 *St. Elizabeth Medical Center: 125 Years of Caring, 1861–1986*, p. 11.

Rev. Sister Pancratia
Superioress

Top: Sr. Pancratia was superior of the sisters at St. Elizabeth Hospital during the 1910s and 1920s. From: Archives of the Franciscan Sisters of the Poor, Hartwell (Cincinnati), Ohio.

Bishop Ferdinand Brossart was a strong supporter of St. Elizabeth Hospital and was instrumental in the opening of its maternity ward. From: St. Camillus Academy brochure, Archives of the Diocese of Covington.

a nurse was a member of an important medical team was a new thought born in the last years of the 19th century. In addition to the nursing school, the staff doctors requested the establishment of a maternity ward. They believed the ward would greatly reduce infant mortality rates and save expectant mothers the necessity of crossing the Ohio River to have their babies in a hospital.

Change, however, seldom comes without some level of resistance and hardship. In 1917 St. Elizabeth Hospital faced a major threat that had a real chance of putting the hospital out of business. Most interestingly, the force threatening the existence of the hospital came from within. Sometime in early 1917, Sister Aurea Schoeder took over after the death of Sister Michaela Schappert as Mother Superior in charge of St. Elizabeth Hospital. Upon taking charge, Sister Schoeder announced that the hospital would no longer support the nursing school nor would it build a maternity ward. Neither project was supported or encouraged by the original founder of the Sisters of the Poor, Frances Schervier, and therefore must be discontinued.[5]

The reaction of the doctors and nurses working at the hospital was quick and decisive. On August 17, 1917, the entire staff of 19 doctors at

the hospital sent a letter to the Mother Provincial resigning their positions at the hospital effective August 31, if she did not immediately rescind her decision.[6] The letter from the doctors was followed three days later by a similar letter from the nurses on staff also resigning as of midnight August 31. The letter was written by Catherine Quinn, superintendent of nurses, and signed by 16 other nurses.[7]

On August 23, Sister Pancratia Sanders, provincial vicar of the order, responded to the doctors at the hospital by stating that the nursing school would remain open, but she could not guarantee that it would be open forever, since she was subject to a higher authority. As for the maternity ward, she wrote that the "Mother House under the protection of the highest Ecclesiastical Authorities, strenuously opposes."[8] The doctors decided to take what victory they could, thanked the sister for her letter, and sought to find a solution to the maternity ward controversy. They worked to make arrangements with Bethesda Hospital to handle St. Elizabeth's birthing needs, but they did not give up on their plan for a ward at St. Elizabeth Hospital in the future.

The doctors just took their quest to another arena. On January 19, 1919, Sister Pancratia

5 Unpublished letter from Mother Provincial to the Bishop of Covington, dated January 15, 1919, in the Sisters of the Poor of St. Francis archive at Hartwell, Ohio.

6 Unpublished letter to Mother Provincial (Sister Pancratia) from 19 doctors on staff at St. Elizabeth Hospital dated August 17, 1917, in the Sisters of the Poor of St. Francis archive at Hartwell, Ohio.

7 Unpublished letter to Mother Provincial from 16 nurses at St. Elizabeth Hospital dated August 20, 1917, in the Sisters of the Poor of St. Francis archive at Hartwell, Ohio.

8 Unpublished letter from Mother Provincial (Sister Pancratia) to the Esteemed Doctors, August 23, 1917, in the Sisters of the Poor of St. Francis archive at Hartwell, Ohio.

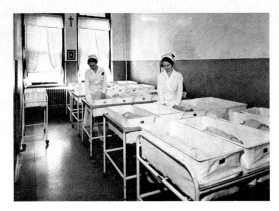

Nursery at St. Elizabeth Hospital, 1935.
From: *Diamond Jubilee: St. Elizabeth's Hospital* (1935).

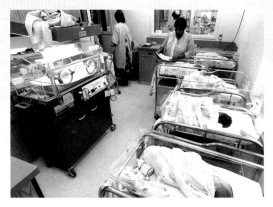

Nursery at St. Elizabeth Hospital, Covington, 1978.
From: St. Elizabeth Healthcare.

Cost of baby in 1932

Bill to Mrs. Chester Geaslen, May 6, 1932

Costs of delivering a baby in 1932 at St. Elizabeth Hospital:

Cost of hospital stay May 5 to May 12, 1932	$20.00
Delivery	$10.00
Medicine and Supplies	$7.00
Total	**$37.00**

Special note:
Bills are payable weekly. Please do not pay by check.

once again received a letter. This time it was from Bishop Ferdinand Brossart of Covington. He strongly suggested that the good sister move forward on the establishment of a permanent obstetrical ward at St. Elizabeth Hospital. Among the many reasons he cited was the forcing of Catholic mothers to have children in non-Catholic hospitals where children may die without the benefit of baptism. He further stated that nurses in the hospital's own nursing school had to complete their training in non-Catholic hospitals since maternity training was required by the state board of nurses. The Bishop politely added that if it was not within her power to do so, to whom could he write to in order move the project forward?[9]

Sister Pancratia's response to the Bishop was similar to her earlier response to the doctors. She argued that the addition of the maternity ward would be a violation of the founding ideals of Mother Frances. She agreed, however, to take the matter to the leaders of her order for further discussion, begging the Bishop's patience in the matter.[10] The challenge it seems was that Sister Pancratia, in her capacity as vicar general, needed approval to open the maternity ward from the superior general located in Germany. The war made such communications almost impossible.[11]

This was not the answer the Bishop was looking for. His next letter was blunt and to the point. The Prefect of the Congregation for Religious at the Vatican, he wrote, had transmitted to him the "rescript" by which the Holy Father kindly deigned, in an audience given the prefect on February 4, 1919, that St. Elizabeth Hospital would open a maternity ward immediately.[12] In other words, the leadership in Rome had superseded the objections of the Sisters of the Poor and St. Elizabeth Hospital would now have an obstetrical department. Rome's only concession to the sisters was the right to close the ward if another Catholic hospital was built that could handle the birthing duties and the right to hire and fire staff as the sisters saw fit. The maternity ward opened within a few months.

The battle over the nursing school and

9 Unpublished letter from Bishop Ferdinand Brossart, Diocese of Covington, to Mother Provincial (Sister Pancratia), dated January 13, 1919, in the Sisters of the Poor of St. Francis archive at Hartwell, Ohio.

10 Unpublished letter to Bishop Ferdinand Brossart, Diocese of Covington, from Mother Provincial (Sister Pancratia), dated January 15, 1919, in the Sisters of the Poor of St. Francis archive at Hartwell, Ohio.

11 Correspondence between author and Sister Jacinta, archivist at Hartwell, Cincinnati, Ohio, January 27, 2011.

12 Unpublished letter from Bishop Ferdinand Brossart, Diocese of Covington, to Mother Provincial (Sister Pancratia), dated March 31, 1919, the Sisters of the Poor of St. Francis archive at Hartwell, Ohio.

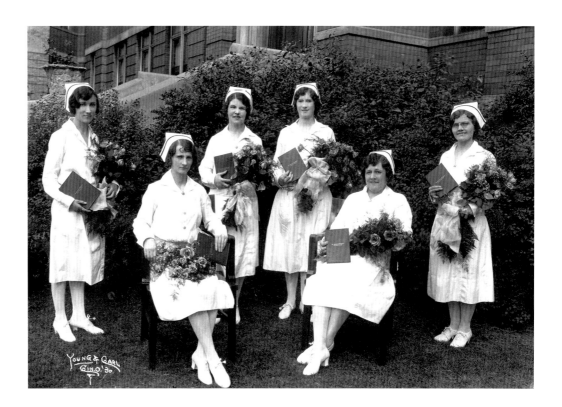

Graduation photo, St. Elizabeth School of Nursing, Covington, May 11, 1930. From: Archives of the Franciscan Sisters of the Poor, Hartwell (Cincinnati), Ohio.

Below: Dr. James Averdick was an influential physician in Covington and Chief of Staff at St. Elizabeth Hospital. From: Michael R. Averdick.

the maternity ward was over but the internal battle between the forces of change and the forces of tradition were far from over. The January 16, 1922, issue of *The Kentucky Post* reported that the sisters managing the hospital once again were closing the nursing school and reorganizing the medical staff, including the removal of Dr. James

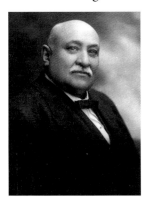

Averdick as chief of staff.[13] It had been Averdick who had written the letter on behalf of the medical staff during the earlier fight for the nursing school. Averdick was a leading physician in the community and was leader of the local Democratic Party. In addition to his dismissal, a number of professionally trained nurses also were discharged. The newspaper further quoted an anonymous

source that the action was taken because the sisters did not like working side by side with nurses who were not of the Order of the Sisters of the Poor of St. Francis. The trouble, according to the newspaper, started when the sisters were forced by the staff doctors and the Catholic clergy to open the maternity ward.

The changes brought on by the internal feud caused an immediate shortage of nurses at the hospital. Many of the nurses who had been fired quickly found jobs in other area hospitals, including 12 who went

to Speers Hospital in Dayton, Kentucky.[14] Leaders at St. Elizabeth may have regretted their move, perhaps not seeing the full impact of their action. They had successfully killed the nursing school, withdrawing their support by not giving the students the lectures and classes that they needed to complete their training. They did this, according to one source, in hope that the students would get frustrated and go

13 "Sisters Nurses – Outsiders Not Wanted at St. Elizabeth," *Kentucky Post*, January 16, 1922, p. 1.

14 *Kentucky Post*, January 25, 1922.

elsewhere, allowing management to close the school. Perhaps regretting her actions, Mother Superior Schoeder offered to reopen the nursing school for three months in order to allow the students to finish their lessons, thus easing the nursing shortage somewhat. The nursing students refused the offer, leaving the doctors at St. Elizabeth to do their own surgical dressings.[15] The sisters' victory was short-lived; the nursing school reopened in 1927.[16]

Despite the internal conflict within St. Elizabeth, the city of Covington's love affair with the hospital continued. The annual report for 1926 reported that 618 babies were born to 606 mothers in the hospital's maternity ward. Obviously, the hospital was so popular with babies that the newspaper reported that some were coming in pairs. In addition to the babies, 3,721 patients were treated in the hospital and 1,092 were treated with first aid and released. Of those treated for first aid, 872 were men and 220 were women. The paper explained that this discrepancy was due to the fact that men "had more hazardous occupations than women, and therefore are more liable to be injured than women."[17] No comment was

15 *Kentucky Post*, January 25, 1922.

16 *Kentucky Post*, February 3, 1927.

17 *Kentucky Post*, January 15, 1927.

Handmade dolls were given to young patients, circa 1950. From: St. Elizabeth Healthcare.

made as to whether men are more accident prone then women.

By 1930, the leadership of St. Elizabeth Hospital fully embraced the training school for nurses. Although there were only six graduates, a ceremony took place at St. Mary's Cathedral in Covington. The class selected the American Beauty rose as the class flower, starting a tradition that would be shared with other graduates for the remaining years of the school. There were 13 graduates in 1932, and 19 graduates in 1934, as the popularity of the school increased. The school continued to grow even through the Depression as money and opportunities became limited for most Americans. At this difficult time in our nation's history, the nursing profession offered steady work for women in a world still dominated by men.

Nurses who graduated from St. Elizabeth Nursing School were taught not only fine nursing skills, but also high moral and ethical standards in keeping with the teachings of the Catholic Church. A 1957 copy of the *Moral Handbook of Nursing* instructed students how to perform many important duties, including how to set up a temporary altar for communion and how to perform an emergency baptism when a priest was

unavailable.[18] In addition to moral and religious instruction, women attending the nursing school were taught how to address doctors, walk straight and upright, and how to keep their uniforms starched and white. Being a successful nurse had much to do with self-discipline.

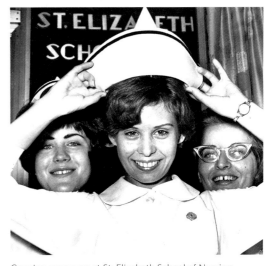

Capping ceremony at St. Elizabeth School of Nursing, Covington. Left to right: Elaine Weber; Betty Hunter; and Rosalie Hurm. From: Kenton County Public Library, Covington.

The crowning achievement for the nursing student was the receiving of her cap upon graduation. The cap indicated that one was now a nurse and no longer a student. A dark stripe across the top of the cap indicated the nursing school

18 Hayes, Edward J., Paul J. Hayes and Dorothy Ellen Kelly, RN, *Moral Handbook of Nursing: a Compendium of Principles, Spiritual Aids and Concise Answers regarding Catholic Personnel, Patients and Problems*, (New York: The Macmillan Company, 1957).

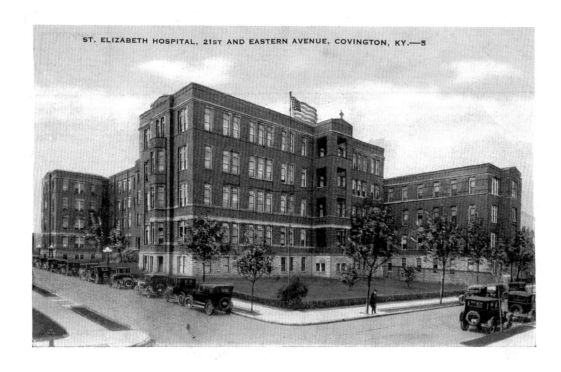

ST. ELIZABETH HOSPITAL, 21ST AND EASTERN AVENUE, COVINGTON, KY.—5

Postcard view of St. Elizabeth Hospital on 20th Street, circa 1937. From: Paul A. Tenkotte, Ph.D.

Right: Staff and Franciscan Sisters of the Poor working in the kitchen of St. Elizabeth Hospital on 20th St., 1935. In addition to serving its patients and staff, the hospital operated a soup kitchen for the poor during the Great Depression. From: *Diamond Jubilee: St. Elizabeth's Hospital* (1935).

Opposite: Flood waters from the Licking River surrounded St. Elizabeth Hospital on 20th St. in 1937. From: *One Hundred Twenty-Five: St. Elizabeth Medical Center* (1986).

in a strict nursing school who triumph over adversity and a tough headmistress to become professional nurses.

The coming of the Great Depression brought tough times to the nation, Northern Kentucky and St. Elizabeth Hospital. The sisters at the hospital had seen tough times before during the Civil War, during the financial crisis of the early years on 11th Street, and during the smallpox and influenza epidemics of previous decades. History seemed to repeat itself as babies were once again left at the hospital, and the institution had more patients who were unable to pay. The hospital's 1933 annual report stated that nearly 70 percent of the patients

from which one graduated. St. Elizabeth's cap had a narrow black stripe at the top of the brim. To many, this was a special source of pride. The nurses' caps used at St. Elizabeth Hospital were of a unique design. The cap came to a point, which rose out of the center of the hat. To nurses and some children in the hospital, the cap reminded them of a witch's hat with the brim cut down. Rumor had it they were designed to duplicate the caps worn by nurses in the 1934 movie *The White Parade* starring Loretta Young.[19] The story is about students

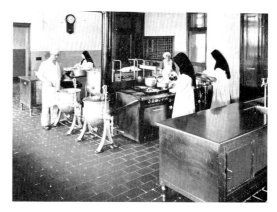

treated at the hospital were treated free of charge.[20] In addition, St. Elizabeth Hospital added a new function to meet the needs of the local community. In September 1931, the hospital opened a soup kitchen which

19 The movie was nominated for a best picture Oscar in 1934.

20 *Kentucky Post*, January 26, 1934.

served between 600 and 800 unemployed and poor people every day.[21]

As in years past, the sisters and supporters of St. Elizabeth helped pay the bills for such ventures with tag sales, bazaars, dinners, concerts and outright solicitations. However, unlike in decades past, things were different now because St. Elizabeth was the community's hospital. The city of Covington gave $10,000 and Kenton County gave $5,000 as annual allotments in support of the hospital's efforts. The votes in the city council and county board were unanimous and no public dissent was noted by the *Kentucky Post*. How things had changed for St. Elizabeth Hospital.

In 1936, St. Elizabeth celebrated its diamond jubilee by hosting a dinner for 700 and raffling off a 1936 Chevrolet at 10 cents a ticket. A newspaper at the time reported that the hospital was "not only the birth place of 75 percent of our local people, but it was here that the first, longest and most enduring bread line originated in the shadows of the hospital doors, during the dark days of the Great Depression."[22] The sisters, doctors, nurses, staff and supporters of St. Elizabeth Hospital had cause to be proud. Since its initial opening on January 21, 1861, the hospital had served 95,943 patients. Over the organization's 75 years, the

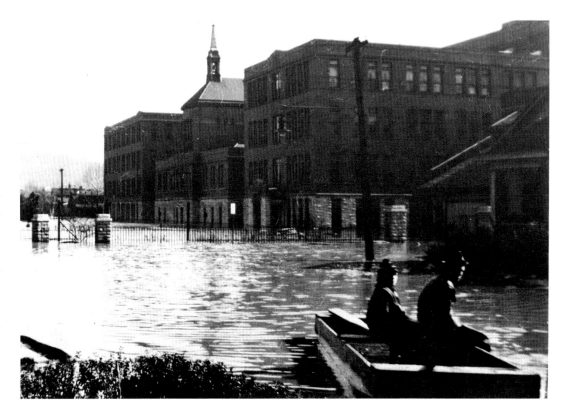

hospital had grown into a thoroughly modern medical organization whose leadership embraced change while keeping the founding principles of caring for all, regardless of religion, ethnic origin or ability to pay.

St. Elizabeth Hospital was never an organization that looked back or rested on its laurels for very long. The institution emerged from its jubilee year with an eye on the future of medicine and the changing needs of the community it served. However, nature had plans for St. Elizabeth Hospital which would tax both the creativity and the

endurance of its staff.

In January 1937, Northern Kentucky suffered the greatest natural disaster in its recorded history. The floodwaters of the Ohio River reached 79.99 feet, which was 27 feet above flood stage. At the height of the disaster 40 percent of the city of Covington was under water, including the basement of St. Elizabeth Hospital. Of the city's residents, 30,000 people were forced from their homes and had to seek shelter elsewhere. St. Elizabeth Hospital became the home for many refugees, including 300

21 *Kentucky Post*, June 14, 1932.

22 *St. Elizabeth Hospital Medical Center: 125 Years of Caring, 1861–1986*, p. 16.

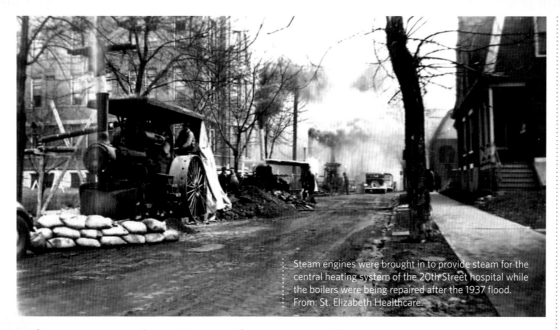

Steam engines were brought in to provide steam for the central heating system of the 20th Street hospital while the boilers were being repaired after the 1937 flood. From: St. Elizabeth Healthcare.

The Battle for the Boilers

The war began on Thursday, January 21, 1937. On one side were men and great machines battling with iron, steel, steam, sinew and sweat. On the other side was the worst storm in decades, with flooded rivers swollen from melting snows ready to show modern humans the folly of their attempt to tame Mother Nature.

The first call to the Covington Fire Department came mid-day that Thursday. The 248 patients at St. Elizabeth Hospital were at risk of losing their heat, and if anything could be done, the 104-year-old Covington Fire Department had the equipment to save the day. Fire Chief Frank Northcutt sent his four best pumpers. The goal was to keep the hospital's basement and sub-basement pumped dry, protecting the hospital's storage of food and the building's brand new $25,000 boilers. Mr. Heck, the hospital's chief maintenance engineer,

directed the work of the fire department. In Heck's opinion, the boilers were his finest achievement in his long career as chief engineer of the hospital. He had worked hard to get the hospital board to buy the boilers, and he had supervised every step of their installation. He would not surrender them to the rising waters of the Ohio River.

But the water kept coming. Thursday became Friday and the fight continued. No one slept and little was eaten by the firefighters or the staff. It was decided that the battle for the sub-basement was lost and all efforts should be shifted to save the boilers in the basement. Before the engines pumping the sub-basement were removed to aid the pumpers working on the boiler room, what food remained in the sub-basement had to be saved. A call to all able-bodied personnel brought a torrent of volunteers, including all student nurses, women

from the office and nurses' aides. The sub-basement was soon emptied of all salvageable food; the room was then abandoned to the rising waters. All efforts were refocused on the boiler room.

But the water kept coming. The fight to save the boilers continued into Saturday, then into Sunday. "Black Sunday," as survivors called it, brought more water and even heavier rains. The call went out for more help, and Hamilton, Ohio, sent two more pumper trucks. By late afternoon the combination of six fire trucks was pumping nearly 2,000 gallons of water out of the boiler room per minute, yet the water was still rising. Heck called for large trucks to dump 50 tons of sand around the base of the building housing the boiler room in hopes to slow the flood waters. By the time the trucks arrived at 5 p.m., the water had almost reached their axles.

But the water kept coming. At 10:30 p.m. Sunday, Chief Northcutt ordered a halt to the effort. There was simply too much water, and now he was at risk of losing his trucks and maybe even his men. The trucks pulled out just in time and had to leave their hoses to the mercy of the rising waters. The waters quickly filled the boiler room, extinguishing the boilers, depriving the hospital of heat. Shortly afterward, the hospital received word that it soon would be without electricity. Darkness and cold were the newest enemies facing the diligent staff. Heck appeared from his battle somehow "older and grayer," saying that God had punished him because he had been too proud of his new boilers.

When the flood waters finally receded and the boiler room was pumped dry nearly a week later, it was found that the boiler room and basement had become the new home of several fish, including a catfish 16 inches long.

This story was pieced together from an unpublished diary entitled "Bird's Eye View and Diary of the Flood of 1937" found in the archives of St. Elizabeth Hospital.

patients already in the hospital. During the flood, the hospital lost both electricity and heat as the water flooded the building's boiler room, despite a gallant effort by staff members and local firefighters.

As an island of refuge in a city of chaos, St. Elizabeth Hospital did what it could for those it could help. Requests came in by boat from people stranded in various locations throughout the city looking for food or supplies, whatever could be spared. The hospital sent out gallons of soup to those in need, including many people trapped in the Kenton County Courthouse. When the waters receded to where vehicles could be safely moved, resourceful staffers at the hospital arranged for a steamroller and steamshovel to be brought to the hospital. The two machines provided the steam needed to heat the hospital, until the building's damaged boilers could be brought back into service.

The next crisis facing the hospital and the people of Northern Kentucky came in the form of a great world war. Like most of the nation, the attack on Pearl Harbor in December 1941 blasted Northern Kentucky and St. Elizabeth out of the Great Depression and into a war footing. War rationing and shortages forced several lay-supporting organizations at the hospital to step up and produce what the hospital could not easily obtain on the market. Items they provided included aprons for orderlies, masks for surgeons, pads and blankets for new babies

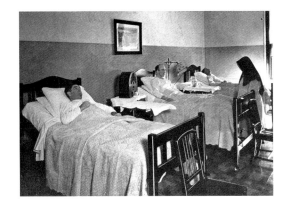

Patients' ward, circa 1935, St. Elizabeth Hospital, Covington. From: *Diamond Jubilee: St. Elizabeth's Hospital* (1935).

and even coverings for bedpans.[23] The volunteer organizations involved in this effort included the Pink Ladies, the Crusaders Club and the Circle of Mercy.

In addition to providing supplies for the war effort and making do with shortages and allowable rations, St. Elizabeth also gave its share of personnel. Doctors, nurses and other employees of the hospital went off to war. Doctors and nurses traded the clean hallways and white uniforms of St. Elizabeth for the often dirty rooms of temporary military hospitals and uniforms of drab olive green. St. Elizabeth never forgot the members of its staff who were serving their country in the military. The hospital erected a plaque in the shape of a V with a blue background and a silver star for each member of the staff who was in the military.[24]

---

23 *St. Elizabeth Hospital Medical Center: 125 Years of Caring, 1861–1986*, p. 17

24 *St. Elizabeth Hospital Medical Center: 125 Years of Caring, 1861–1986*, p. 17.

St. Elizabeth Hospital Finds New Way to "Treat" Visiting "Fakers"

C.M. Fulton was a professional "faker." That is to say he made a living faking illnesses. This allowed him the ability to arouse sympathy and gain access to "treatments" at hospitals. It is said Fulton was especially good at controlling his facial and stomach muscles, thereby putting on a convincing act of being overwhelmed with pain. Whenever he needed a rest, he would fake one of his attacks and be taken to the hospital for free food and relaxation. He did this so often that Covington police gave him the nickname "Fakers."

One Sunday in 1940, "Fakers" was found by police at 33rd Street and Decoursey Avenue rolling in pain. The officers took him to St. Elizabeth Hospital even though they knew him from similar incidents in the weeks before. The staff at the hospital was also aware of his exploits and was not fooled by his act of illness. The nurse on duty approached patient "Fakers" while he wriggled in pain on the examination room table and promptly stuck him in the thigh with a hat pin, which immediately cured him of his illness. The police took the now-cured Mr. Fulton into custody. The next day he was fined $25 in city court.

From the *Kentucky Post*, September 9, 1940

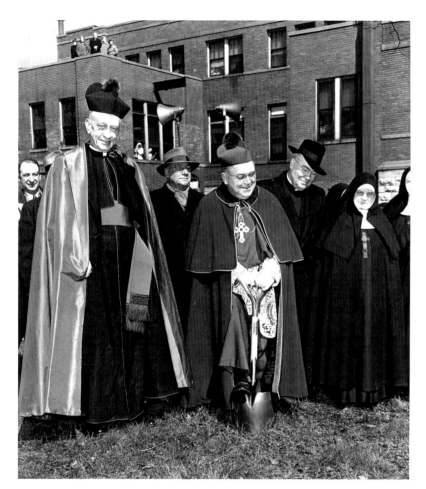

Bishop William Mulloy breaks ground for the new student nurses' residence (Tarsicia Hall), 1949. From: St. Elizabeth Healthcare.

Right: 1974 photo of Earl Gilreath, the first lay administrator of St. Elizabeth Hospital. From: St. Elizabeth Healthcare.

Opposite: In 1967 the Franciscan Sisters added lay members to the Board of Trustees of St. Elizabeth. Left to right: Charles Deters; Sr. Marie Bernard; Dr. William Middendorf; and Gayle McElroy. Sr. Marie Bernard was the last Franciscan Sister of the Poor to serve as administrator of St. Elizabeth Hospital. From: *One Hundred Twenty-Five: St. Elizabeth Medical Center* (1986)

Perhaps it can be argued that the impact of World War II on St. Elizabeth was not in the war effort or in the lives of those from the hospital who served, but rather what came after the war. In 1944, the last full year of the war, the hospital reported 1,439 babies born in the maternity ward. In 1946, the hospital recorded 1,759 babies born, an increase of 320 babies. In 1947, the hospital recorded 2,203 births, including 24 sets of twins, 444 more than the previous year and 764 more than in 1944.[25] The baby boom had hit the maternity ward at St. Elizabeth Hospital.

The late 1940s and early 1950s were periods of great expansion and growth for the hospital. Concerns over polio led to the creation of a children's orthopedic unit in 1946 (funded by the Rotary Clubs of Northern Kentucky) followed soon afterward by a psychiatric unit. In 1950 a home for nursing students (Tarsicia Hall), with a capacity for 200 nurses, was completed at a cost of $800,000.[26]

In the 1960s, the Sisters of the Poor of St. Francis, who had managed the hospital from the beginning, began to see that time was beginning to catch up with them. The leadership in the form of the board of trustees and the administrator of the hospital had always been the Sisters of the Poor. Dwindling numbers of women were joining the order, making it more difficult to manage the

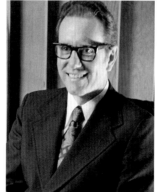

hospital's affairs. In 1962 the sisters decided that creating an advisory board of lay community leaders to help make important decisions was necessary. The sisters were still capable administrators, but they recognized that the hospital was now a business.

In 1967 it became clear to the Sisters of the Poor that they could no longer manage the hospital and that they needed some other organization to take

25 St. Elizabeth Hospital annual reports for 1944–1947.

26 Mother Tarsicia Marie had reorganized the hospital's school of nursing.

over. The biggest concern of the sisters was that the hospital maintain its dedication to the poor and to the Catholic principles it supported. The logical choice was the Diocese of Covington. In 1968 the sisters officially transferred management of the hospital to the diocese, which appointed St. Elizabeth's first lay and first male administrator, Earl Gilreath.[27]

Prior to Gilreath's appointment, and only a few months after a board of trustees composed of both religious and lay board members was established, the hospital faced a new crisis. In November 1967, the nurses at St. Elizabeth Hospital threatened to strike over issues of salary, working conditions and the right to collective bargaining. The new board was open to negotiating the issues of salary and working conditions at the hospital, but not on the issue of allowing the nurses to form a union. On November 16, as communications between the nurses and the administration became strained, some nurses walked off their jobs, leaving the hospital shorthanded. Mother Mary Julian stepped forward as a liaison between the hospital and the nurses, as she was trusted by both parties.

Because St. Elizabeth Hospital had become such an important part of the community, the strike was big news. Community opinion ran freely in both directions.

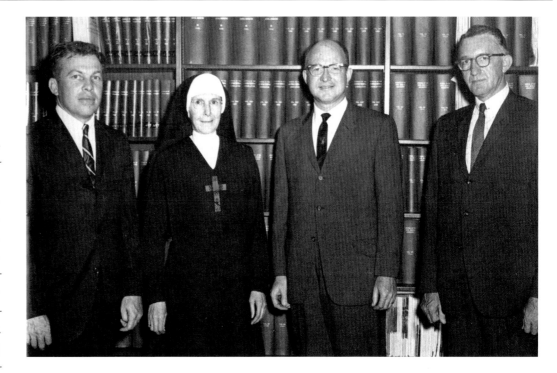

Some citizens referred to the striking nurses in derogatory terms, while others saw them as crusaders for justice and quality care for hospital patients. Even the mayor of Covington, Bernard F. Eicholz, supported the nurses and urged the St. Elizabeth board of trustees to recognize the nurses' right to collective bargaining through the Registered Nurses Organization. The nurses were also supported by nurses at St. Luke Hospital in Fort Thomas. The strike ended after the hospital recognized the nurses' right to collective bargaining. The nurses returned to their jobs.

During the strike, an incident occurred that revealed the dedicated nature of the

nurses, despite their conflict with the board. On November 20, 1967, Trans World Airlines flight 126 crashed during an attempted landing at the Greater Cincinnati Airport (now called the Cincinnati/Northern Kentucky International Airport). As the first alarm after the crash was sounded, many of the striking nurses at St. Elizabeth Hospital ignored the walkout and returned to work. The dedication of these nurses to those in need would have made the sisters who founded the first St. Elizabeth extremely proud. The incident revealed the commitment that these fine citizens had to their community and to their profession. They were there when they were needed,

27 *St. Elizabeth Hospital Medical Center: 125 Years of Caring, 1861-1986*, pp. 20-21.

November 20, 1967, TWA Flight 126

by Don Clare, Nurse

It was a Monday evening and I had just arrived at my girlfriend's house for a visit. We were sitting on the couch and the local evening news was on the TV reporting that there had been an airliner crash at the Greater Cincinnati Airport. The wreckage was strewn all over a Hebron farmer's orchard somewhere on the approach of the intended runway. I remember that it was pretty cold and there had been either fine mist or snow flurries requiring windshield wipers, but nothing accumulating.

At the time, my mother had been an assistant director of nurses at St. Elizabeth Hospital in Covington, and she had not been home at all the previous week because there had been a nurses' strike going on for about a week. She was virtually living at the hospital and working with the other supervisors, taking care of the patients and keeping the hospital running. I remember some of the other supervisors being Dorothy Fite, Gloria Ferkenhoff, and my mother. It seems like the nurses had organized a similar strike as the one that had just recently taken place in Detroit hospitals. They were requesting a fairer wage and more adequate equipment in order to deliver better patient care.

When I heard the news that the injured were being transported to St E's, I decided to drive down there to see if I could be of any help to my mother and the others who were going to be receiving all these victims. There was no idea of how many injured would be showing up, or how many dead there were, but you quickly got the feeling that things were bound to be ugly.

When I arrived, I remember walking in the main entrance doors and up those very ornate steps to the main floor, where the chapel was prominently located. Immediately, I ran into my mother, who was right there in the hall in an impromptu conference with other nurses, all wearing their white dresses, stockings, shoes and their nursing caps. They were busily planning strategies for this impending disaster. (I don't even know if hospitals had disaster plans back then, but there was certainly one in the making, with drawings, maps, sketches and the like.)

I remember she didn't even greet me. She looked up and saw me and promptly said, "Don, you go down to the emergency room (which literally was just a room) on the backside of the building near the courtyard and the stone archway entrance doors to the ground floor."

The scene was congestion and utter, but organized, chaos. There were ambulances and hearses pulling in and unloading stretchers. I reported to the person (a man) who appeared to be taking charge of the chaos but in reality was triaging (before that term was popular in the private sector). I told him who I was and he assigned me to assist some other folks in what turned out to be the morgue section. My job was to gather belongings and valuables and put them in what I think were interoffice mail envelopes and lay them on the person with some kind of notation. Truthfully, to this very day, the only real recollections of that night were my being there and attending to my duties and the overwhelming smell of jet fuel. Everything and everybody smelled of it.

The night is all a blur to me now, conveniently and no doubt deliberately suppressed somewhere into the very back of my mind. I still retain just a few vivid memories. One was my arrival and seeing my mother's face and making eye contact with her without really getting to converse. Another was the feeling of hope and relief as all the striking nurses began showing up and taking charge and doing the things nurses do—taking care of the immediate physical and emotional needs of the injured and dying. It was like "the strike be damned, let's relieve the pain and suffering of these unfortunate people." There was just a steady din and cacophony of moaning, crying, screaming, hysteria. It now all seems so surreal. The pungent odor of jet fuel is a very lasting memory.

Overall, there were 14 survivors taken to St. Elizabeth; three taken to Booth (also in Covington); and one taken to General Hospital in Cincinnati (now University).

Virginia Clare was a longtime Assistant Director of Nursing at St. Elizabeth on 20th St. She was supervisor of nurses at the time of the 1967 crash of TWA Fight 128 at the Greater Cincinnati Airport. A former teacher at Good Counsel School, she was among the recipients of the Outstanding Women of Northern Kentucky of 1995. She also served on the Board of Trustees of St. Elizabeth. From: Don Clare.

continuing a St. Elizabeth legacy for more than 100 years. As the saying goes, "Nurses are angels in comfortable shoes." Some survivors of the plane crash still keep in touch with the St. Elizabeth nurses that cared for them. One passenger who was severely injured returned to witness the graduation of the student nurses who cared for her when she was recuperating from the accident.

Earl Gilreath's legacy as chief executive officer of St. Elizabeth Hospital was one of expansion and construction. During his tenure, St. Elizabeth on 20th Street underwent a major renovation and new construction. The nursing school closed as nurses' training shifted to colleges and universities, and the building was renovated into more patient rooms, and a state-of-the-art emergency room was added. In 1972 the first total hip replacement in Northern Kentucky was performed at St. Elizabeth, followed a year later by the first total knee replacement. In 1973 the maternity department started a revolutionary program to allow fathers in the delivery room during birth.

One of the lasting practices of St. Elizabeth Hospital is its administrators' propensity for responding to the needs of the community. The hospital did so on the day it established its first building in

Top: Childbirth class, circa 1970s. From: St. Elizabeth Healthcare.

Right: Aerial view of St. Elizabeth Hospital South, Edgewood. From: Kenton County Public Library, Covington.

Covington in 1861. It did it again with the opening of new facilities on 11th and 20th streets, as well as the creation of the nursing school, and the maternity ward. Then, in anticipation of the growth and shift in population brought by the I-75 and I-275 freeways, hospital administrators turned their attention south and west. In the late 1960s, the hospital invested in 260 acres in Edgewood, with plans to build a medical center in the region that was second to none. This new facility would be called the South Unit. The hospital in Covington would be referred to as the North Unit. The genius of building St. Elizabeth Hospital

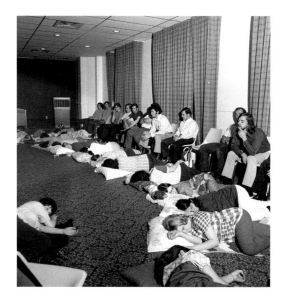

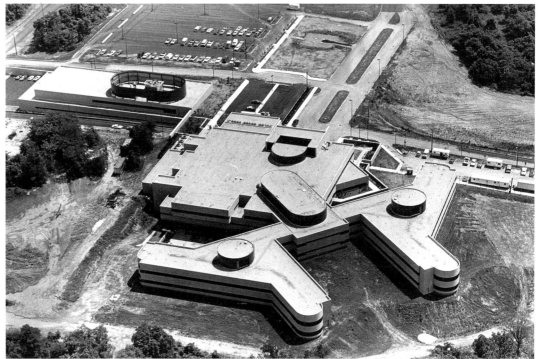

"Every Time We Did Something Well, More Patients Came"

Joseph W. Gross, St. Elizabeth Healthcare President and Chief Executive Officer, 1986–2010

"A great Monday" was the simple but profound way Joseph Gross described the day he walked into his Edgewood office and learned that St. Elizabeth had been named a "Top 100" U.S. hospital. Could the explanation equally be as simple as "every time we did

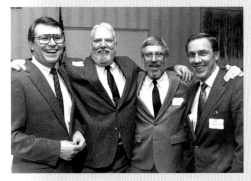

Left to right: Joe Gross, administrator from 1986 until 2010; Dr. Andy Baker; Dr. Ron Lubbe; and Dr. John Darpel. From: St. Elizabeth Healthcare.

something well, more patients came"? Most people who have watched St. Elizabeth grow from "a diamond in the rough" to the regional leader it is today would credit the role Joe Gross himself played in the transformation.

And yet, despite emphasizing with an emphatic table thump that he wanted "generations looking back on this generation to know that the patient care they ... depend on ... started here and now," Gross reflects with modest pride on what he

considers his proudest moments at St. Elizabeth's helm. In addition to the quality awards that have rained down in recent years, Gross cites St. Elizabeth employees voting it as a great place to work, the ground-breaking and lifesaving care of patients, and a merger with St. Luke's, which was achieved with "nobody losing their job."

According to Gross, the secret lies in people. "Our product is health care and the raw material is people ... selfless ... people who have chosen this work when they could have [chosen] something much more spectacular ... [usually] for reasons that are bigger than themselves ... they have chosen to work in this non-profit atmosphere." He continues by noting that in the evaluations that led to the awarding of the Magnet designation for nursing, a phrase kept appearing: St. Elizabeth was "one big family." A family caring for a larger family—the Northern Kentucky community—is a major reason that St. Elizabeth has become "part of the bedrock of this community and a key ingredient that keeps the community together." In Joe Gross's eyes, the humble venture started by "those brave nuns" has become "a common gold thread throughout our community."

in Edgewood was the ability it offered for continued growth to meet the needs of an ever-expanding medical profession. At one time, the focus of medicine was the treatment of illness. But now medicine had changed to see the patient more holistically and treat not only their diseases but also their causes and prevention.

The adoption of this new philosophy of healthcare brought a new name to St. Elizabeth Hospital: St. Elizabeth Medical Center. St. Elizabeth now had two centers, the North Unit in Covington and the South Unit in Edgewood. By the time the South Unit opened, St. Elizabeth had a new Chief Executive Officer, Paul Bellendorf. Edgewood was Bellendorf's legacy, and much of the expansion and the innovations over the next few decades were the result of the hard work and planning by him and his leadership team. The expansion and the planning did not come without controversy. Other hospitals in the area objected to the expansions and attempted to derail St. Elizabeth's plans with lawsuits and legislation.[28]

The next Chief Executive Officer of St. Elizabeth, Joseph W. Gross, assumed leadership in 1986 and inherited an organization that was striving to meet the needs of its ever-changing community. Fortunately for Gross, the legacy of the Sisters of the Poor, and Gilreath and Bellendorf had left a medical health business that had the necessary tools to do the job. But, like a good sea captain who looks beyond the smooth seas, ahead to opportunities beyond the horizon, Gross was a man of vision. Gross sold the board of trustees an image not only of a medical center that met the needs of the community it served, but also of a hospital organization that could be a national leader in the field of modern medicine. St. Elizabeth could not only be a leader in Northern Kentucky, but also recognized as one of the top healthcare centers in the United States.

In 1993 St. Elizabeth Hospital acquired Grant County Hospital in Williamstown, Kentucky. This small but mighty hospital had its humble beginnings as a 30-room facility started in 1964. One of the principal community leaders responsible for the founding of

---

28 *Kentucky Post*, September 8, 1982.

the hospital was Doris Vest Clark, an executive with the DuBois Chemical Company, one of the few females to hold such a position in America at the time. She also served as a Captain in the Women's Air Corps, WAC, during World War II.[29] Clark was a prominent, no-nonsense community leader who served on numerous boards, including the Grant County Chamber of Commerce and the American Red Cross.

It is therefore no surprise that the hospital that she helped found soon earned the reputation as the little hospital that could. By the time St. Elizabeth Healthcare had taken over management of Grant County Hospital in 1993, Grant County had almost doubled in population from 18,898 in 1960 to nearly 30,000 in 1990. A growing community needs a hospital to meet a variety of new challenges. The hospital offers many services, including sophisticated cancer treatments, cardiology, urology, emergency medicine, and orthopedic care. Especially notable is St. Elizabeth Grant County's commitment to heart attack victims. The little hospital has received national recognition for its ability to get a heart attack patient prepared and ready for transport to a larger hospital where emergency procedures can be performed—faster than any other hospital of its size. During a heart attack, time is critical to heart muscle, so the longer it takes to get proper care to the patient, the longer recovery will be. In this case, minutes really do count.

CEO Joseph Gross had laid the ground work for the hospital's major expansions. According to

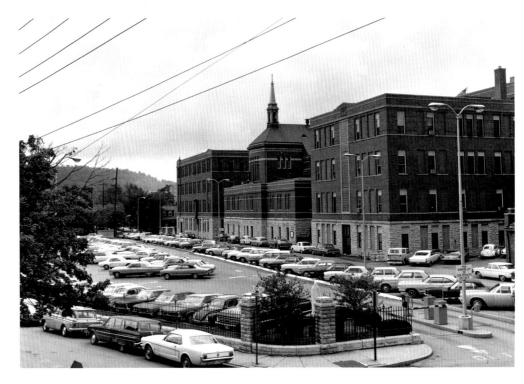

Gross, the pieces of the puzzle were all there: the people, the facilities, the community support and a leadership team that could capture the vision. Despite this, not all hospital associates were sold on the idea. Gross recalled in a 2010 interview that once the plans for the future were announced, he was approached by someone who objected to the vision. The person told him, "I see what you are trying to do, and I am going to fight you every inch of the way." Years later, the same person approached him and sheepishly confessed that Gross had been right all along.[30]

St. Elizabeth Hospital, 20th St., circa early 1970s. From: photo by Raymond E. Hadorn in the collection of Paul A. Tenkotte, Ph.D.

Emergency room nurses, 20th St., 1968, Willie Meehan and Christina Seeger. From: St. Elizabeth Healthcare.

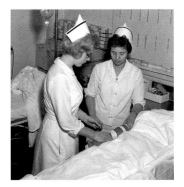

29 *Encyclopedia of Northern Kentucky*, p. 196.

30 Interview with Joseph Gross, CEO St. Elizabeth Healthcare, conducted by Rebecca Bailey, Ph. D., Northern Kentucky University, September 2010.

"We Identify Ourselves by Our Actions"

Terry Foster, Emergency Nurse

To work in a faith-based institution like St. Elizabeth is special to today's associates but no one expresses it more movingly than emergency nurse, Terry Foster. Starting as a teen volunteer in the early 1970s, Foster was hired as a ward clerk, received training as an LPN and finally earned his RN credentials in the late 1970s. Always drawn to "challenges" and possessing a consciousness of how St. Elizabeth herself "cared for the poor, the elderly and socially outcast," Foster chose to specialize in emergency and intensive care.

The possibility of losing patients does not diminish Foster's love of his "divine assignment," as he observes, "Maybe I can't save that patient's life, but I can make sure they have a dignified and peaceful death." Memories of his patients stay with him, but he takes comfort in a commitment that has motivated St. Elizabeth's associates since the good nuns first came to Covington. Day-to-day work in the ER involves

"taking care of ... old people, poor people, somebody from the jail, or a prisoner ... or some person ... who has no one in this world who knows anything about them, or loves them, or cares for them ... and my presence [may be] the last thing ... [they remember] as they leave this world."

Why would Foster find solace and even take pride in caring for people "even the jail won't take"? It comes back to faith and hope. Like the nuns in whose footsteps he follows, Foster finds inspiration in this saying of Jesus Christ: "Whatsoever you do to the least of my people, you do unto me." Hope also motivates Foster because "someday, if my family can't be there, maybe somebody [else] will be, for me."

Foster opens his story with the observation "that it used to be that people would say if you needed medical care, crawl, drive, do whatever you have to do to get across the river to Cincinnati," but that the situation is "absolutely opposite now." As Terry Foster's story illustrates, cutting-edge technology and superior clinical care are not the only components in the equation of success and growth. The other ingredient may be harder to quantify, but it is no less tangible. St. Elizabeth associates enfold those they serve in loving compassion.

The latest crowning achievement in the history of St. Elizabeth was the merger with Northern Kentucky's other great healthcare system, St. Luke. At one time St. Luke and St. Elizabeth hospitals were in competition. Both organizations were made up of highly skilled doctors, nurses, professional staff members and leadership teams with vision. Conversations that began quietly and earnestly between members of the two organizations' leaders culminated in a merger in 2008. St. Elizabeth Vice President of Medical Affairs, Dr. George Hall credits the hard work of Gross and John S. Dubis with the success of the merger.[31] Hall, at the time, was on the board of St. Luke Hospital and was one of the first approached when the idea of a merger surfaced.

With the merger of the two medical care systems, the resulting new organization became St. Elizabeth Healthcare. Still affiliated with the Diocese of Covington, the new hospital system is made up of six major facilities and numerous satellite facilities designed to meet the needs of the community from the treatment of diabetes to substance abuse. The merger also created the opportunity to establish a large hospital-owned multi-disciplinary physicians organization that included two large established physician practices, Patient First and Summit. Formed as St. Elizabeth Physicians in January 2010, the organization now boasts 200 physicians and 50 mid-level providers. St. Elizabeth Physicians specialties include: cardiology, endocrinology, family medicine, gastroenterology, general surgery, internal medicine, neurology, obstetrics/gynecology, pediatrics, pulmonology, and rheumatology. The hospital and physician group merger resulted in the creation of Northern Kentucky's largest employer with over 7,300 employees and over two million square feet of medical facilities in Boone, Campbell, Grant, Kenton and Pendleton counties.[32]

31 Interview with Dr. George Hall conducted by Rebecca Bailey, Ph. D., Northern Kentucky University, December 2010.

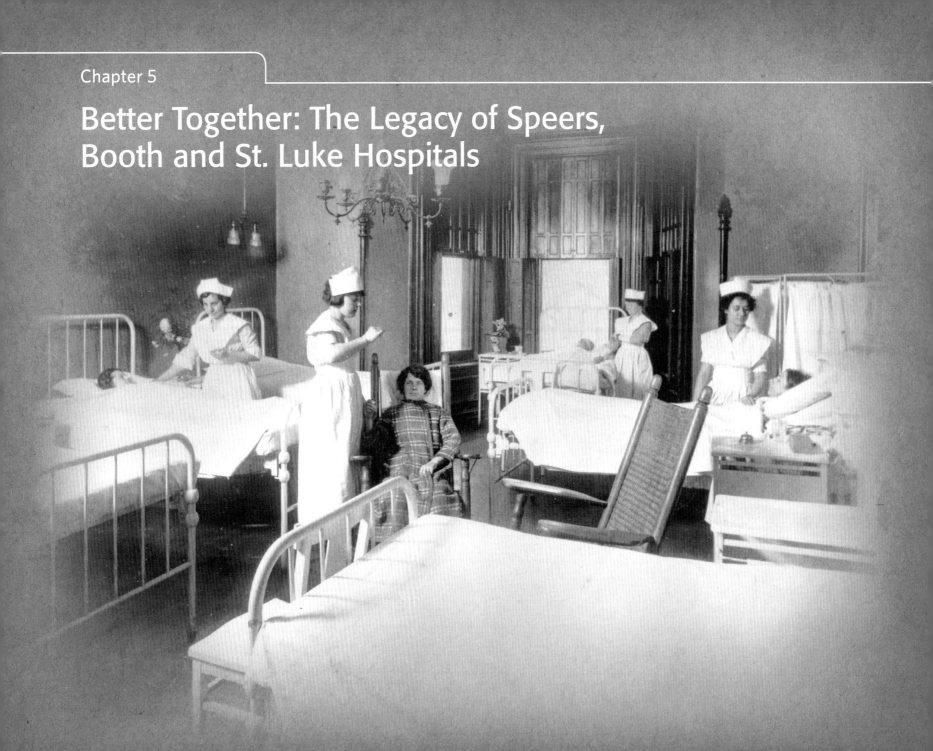

Chapter 5

Better Together: The Legacy of Speers, Booth and St. Luke Hospitals

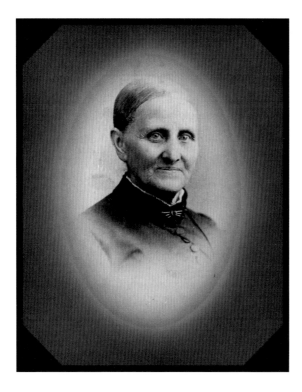

The merger that created St. Elizabeth Healthcare was more than a combination of St. Luke and St. Elizabeth. Part of the legacy that made up these two great hospitals is found in the shadows of other great hospitals, their staffs and the communities that they served. To understand the important building blocks that created the uniqueness of Northern Kentucky's largest employer and one of America's finest healthcare systems, it is important to understand these other institutions.

Speers Memorial Hospital, Dayton, Kentucky

Two hallmarks distinguish Speers Memorial Hospital: financial instability and a dogged determination to stay alive. When Elizabeth Speers passed away in August 1894 in her adopted hometown of Dayton, Kentucky, her funeral was a grand affair. Bells rang all over the city and the local newspaper reported that her funeral was one of the largest anyone in the town had ever seen.[1] The real surprise came when Elizabeth's will was read and it was announced

1 Reis, Jim. "Wealthy Widow's Gift leads to Campbell's First Hospital," *Kentucky Post*, December 21, 1998. See also: Alvin C. Poweleit and James A. Schroer, editors, *A Medical History of Campbell and Kenton Counties* (Campbell-Kenton County Medical Society, ca. 1970); and Alvin C. Poweleit and James A. Schroer, editors, *Medical History of Northern Kentucky* (Northern Kentucky Medical Society, ca. 1989).

that she had left the citizens of Dayton a gift in the form of a hospital named in honor of her husband, Charles C. Speers.

Charles Speers had made a fortune just outside of Houston, Texas, growing cotton and owning slaves. The 1860 Slave Census of the federal government reports that Speers owned 25 enslaved humans ranging in age from 45 years to six months.[2] Sometime after the Civil War, he moved to Cincinnati and later to Dayton, Kentucky, where he died in 1885.

The $100,000 that Mrs. Speers left to the hospital was under the control of three trustees: John Trapp, Charles Nagel and Dr. C.B. Schoolfield. Work began on what was to become Speers Memorial Hospital in the fall of 1895. The new hospital occupied the entire block between Main and Boone streets and Forth and Fifth streets and cost $75,000 to build.[3] When completed, Speers Hospital was four stories tall with 32 rooms and a capacity of 70 patients. One of the most striking features was a life-size statue of Elizabeth Speers cut from Italian marble.[4] Speers Hospital opened on October 1, 1897. A newspaper article boasted that the hospital had indoor bathrooms, private rooms, open wards for multiple patients and an operating room "said to be the finest in the United States."[5]

However, just three years later, the *Kentucky Post* on August 4, 1900, announced that the hospital would close for financial reasons. Nagel told the newspaper that almost since the opening of the hospital, it had been a victim of "ignorant prejudice" from townspeople and doctors who refused to send their patients to Speers. He added that the hospital would be closed for three years in order to show the people of the community how badly they needed a hospital.[6] Two weeks later, the same paper reported that the medical staff at Speers had met with Dayton Mayor Nelson in hopes of coming up with a plan to keep the hospital open. The doctors were concerned not only for their patients but also because the hospital had contracts with the cities of Dayton, Newport and Bellevue for the care of indigents which already had been paid.[7]

The plan developed by the doctors and the mayor was to increase the size of the board of trustees. The circuit court judge

2 1860 U.S. Federal Census—Slave Schedules, City of Houston, County of Harris, Texas, p. 27.

3 *Encyclopedia of Northern Kentucky*, p. 847.

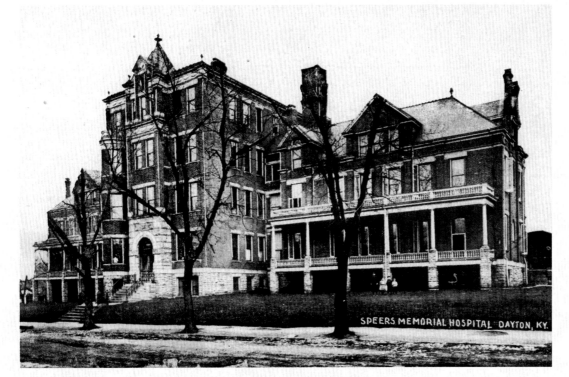

SPEERS MEMORIAL HOSPITAL DAYTON, KY.

4 "CP" August 19, 1896, p. 2.

5 *Kentucky Post*, August 27, 1897, p. 1.

6 *Kentucky Post*, August 5, 1900, p. 5.

7 *Kentucky Post*, August 17, 1900, p. 5.

appointed four new trustees bringing the total to five after Nagel and Trapp resigned in protest of the judge's appointment of new trustees. All the new appointees, including the last remaining original member of the board, were physicians on staff at Speers Hospital.[8] The new board wasted no time to change the financial situation at

the hospital and to improve services. The first step was to appoint Cora Amann as the new superintendent of the hospital and to set up a fundraiser in the form of a dinner and euchre competition at the hospital.[9] The trustees further decided that the hospital needed trained nurses. The result of this decision was the creation of the Speers nurses training school in May 1901.

A year later, the young hospital was in

trouble and once again threatened to close. The hospital was losing money at the rate of approximately $100 a month. As a result, it sought aid from local governments, who reluctantly agreed to increase their payments to the hospital. Finally things seemed to be looking up for Speers Hospital. In 1903 the hospital was finally running in the black and the first class of nurses—seven young women—graduated from the nursing school.

But the good times for Speers did not last long. The very next year, at the commencement ceremony for the new class of graduating nurses, things fell apart. Judge Albert S. Berry, a former Confederate cavalry officer and politician, used the occasion of the nurses' graduation to give a commencement speech blasting the hospital's board of trustees. In his speech to the assembled crowd, he charged the trustees with mismanagement and threatened to remove the board and replace them with business people, not doctors. The judge's next move was to order a grand jury to investigate the hospital and its management. The trustees of the hospital acted quickly and filed a petition against Berry claiming that he had a long-standing personal grudge against the hospital and its board of trustees and could

not be trusted to rule fairly on cases involving the hospital. Further, the petition stated that the judge "has promised several persons to appoint them trustees," before his investigation of the hospital began.[10] Berry refused to even look at the petition and moved forward with the grand jury investigation. Speers had no choice other than to answer the charges in open court.

The judge's attack on the hospital seems to have been primarily motivated by politics and personal greed. Since the founding of the hospital, there were a number of individuals, including relatives of Mrs. Speers, who felt that perhaps they deserved a bigger share of her estate. They saw some of the expenditures of the hospital, including the nursing school, as being an extravagance which used more money than was necessary. One of the other individuals pushing for an investigation was John Trapp, who had resigned in protest from the board of trustees during the first financial crisis. Since then, he had attempted to sue the hospital for "several hundred dollars" in an attempt to force the hospital into receivership.[11] Judge Berry seems to have taken the various malcontents with complaints against the hospital and brought them together for his own purposes, which may have been to appoint political allies to positions of importance at the hospital.

8 *Kentucky Post*, September 29, 1900.

9 *Kentucky Post*, October 2, 1900.

10 *Kentucky Post*, November 12, 1904, p. 1.

11 *Kentucky Post*, November 12, 1904.

The first casualty of the war between the judge and the Speers board of trustees was the hospital superintendent, Cora Amann. In January 1905 she tendered her resignation, citing the stress of the outside litigation combined with the stress of the day-to-day operations of the hospital. The head nurse at the hospital, Sophia Steinhauer, was appointed interim superintendent to replace Amann. Steinhauer would hold the 'temporary" position of superintendent for more than 20 years.

The trustees then went on the attack. First, they denied Judge Berry's jurisdiction in the case, claiming that he had no right to demand a review of the hospital's books or the resignation of the trustees. Secondly, they filed suit against a number of individuals claiming libel. The civil court demurred on the libel cases, stating that although it agreed with the facts of each case, there was insignificant evidence to support the case.[12] The Kentucky Court of Appeals ruled that Judge Berry had no jurisdiction in the case and barred him from further involvement, appointing a special judge, John D. Carroll, to investigate the charges against Speers Hospital.

Carroll's attorneys ordered counsel from both sides to assemble their cases for review, giving them a deadline of nearly a year. After his timeline had passed, the judge issued a contempt of court ruling against attorney Reuscher, lawyer for the individuals suing the hospital, for not having his filings completed. It was a signal from the judge that he would not tolerate the le-

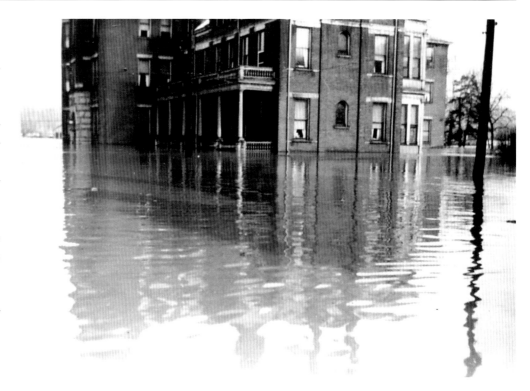

gal maneuvering that was so prominent in Judge Berry's court. Meanwhile, Judge Carroll was replaced by special Judge W. B. Moody, because Judge Carroll had subsequently been appointed to the Kentucky Court of Appeals. In April 1906, Moody ruled in favor of the Speers trustees, stating that there was no proof that the trustees had mismanaged the hospital. He further ruled that the trustees should be commended for the good work they had done and that the plaintiffs in the case, including George Huber and Frank Brinkman, should pay the court costs of the hospital.

With their legal problems over, the trustees of Speers Hospital returned their attention to running a first-rate hospital and finding a way

Flood of 1937 engulfs Speers Hospital. From: Jan D. Stanley.

Opposite: Speers Hospital, 1923. From: Kenton County Public Library, Covington.

---

12 *Kentucky Post,* February 23, 1905, p. 1.

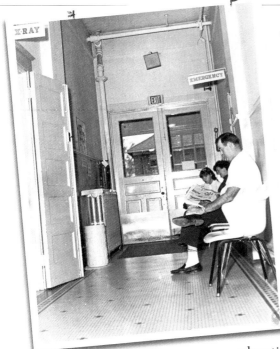

Lobby, Speers Hospital.
From: Kenton County Public Library.

Opposite: Mary Ann Hemingray Shinkle donated her mansion on E. 2nd St., Covington to the Women's Social Department of the New York City branch of the Salvation Army in 1909. It subsequently became the William Booth Memorial Hospital. From: Paul A. Tenkotte, Ph.D.

to pay for it. Financial woes continued even as the hospital sought to expand its services. In 1911 the hospital opened a children's ward with funds donated by the Ladies Aid Society. The opening was well attended with a full orchestra and refreshments served by volunteers.[13] Meanwhile, the nursing school was growing steadily. The program took three years to complete and in 1914, because of improved funding at the hospital, the student nurses were paid while getting their education. All students were given free room and board. In addition, first-year students received $5 a month, second-year students $7 a month and third-year students $10 a month.[14]

Part of the reason for the financial turnaround for the hospital was a contract the hospital had obtained with the Chesapeake and Ohio Railroad to serve as one of the railroad's official hospitals. Under the contract, the hospital would admit sick and injured employees of the railroad as part of the employees' benefits package. Prior to the contract with Speers, employees of the railroad would need to go to West Virginia for treatment. Under the contract, Speers agreed not only to take care of the C&O employees, but also to

maintain an ambulance at the Dayton Depot to transport sick or injured employees to and from the hospital. Because of this contract with the railroad, Speers became known as the "railroaders' hospital."

Despite the temporary reprieve from financial crisis thanks to the contract with the C&O Railroad, the small hospital's money problems continued. In the years 1916, 1928, 1932 and 1937, the hospital sought help from the community, local governments and even the state legislature. Money raised went to pay off debts, remodel the building, build a new boarding house for the ever-popular nursing school and pay for damages after the 1937 flood. The appeal of 1916 even compared the hospital and its mission to be similar to that of St. Elizabeth Hospital in Covington, stating that the hospital had become an essential part of the community, especially serving the poor.[15]

The hospital continued to struggle with financial difficulties even after the Depression. In the late 1940s more than $1 million was raised to build a new hospital in Campbell County that was more centrally located and safe from further floods. The result was the birth of another hospital—St. Luke, in Fort Thomas. Speers Hospital was eventually taken over by St. Elizabeth Hospital in 1973. By then Speers was sadly outdated, and despite a talented and dedicated staff, costs of upgrading the facility were prohibitive. Speers Hospital closed that same year.

13 *Kentucky Post*, June 8, 1911, p. 7.

14 *Kentucky Post*, November 21, 1914, p. 2.

15 *Kentucky Post*, September 27, 1916. p. 1.

Booth Memorial Hospital

Bradford Shinkle was a businessman from a family with wealth. His father was responsible for the building of the Roebling Bridge as president of the Covington and Cincinnati Bridge Company. Bradford had interests in banking, wholesale grocery supply and glass making. He did not drink, smoke or attend social gatherings, preferring to stay at home with his family. He also had a fear of being buried alive, leaving standing orders to have his body watched after his death to assure that he really was dead.[16]

Once it was determined that death had truly come for Bradford Shinkle in 1909, his wife Mary Anne Hemingray Shinkle, moved forward with her plans for the 33-room family home on Second Street in Covington. She donated the house and much of its contents to the Women's Social Department of New York City, a branch of the Salvation Army. The Salvation Army is a Protestant evangelical denomination whose mission is to preach the gospel of Jesus and meet human needs without discrimination. Its organization is based on the framework of a military army with its

ministers and missionaries holding an official rank within the church, such as captain or major.

The Women's Social Department of the Salvation Army was organized by the church to work with matters of concern to women, especially women in need. The organization operated the Shinkle mansion in Covington as a home for young, unmarried women and their newborn babies. It also

operated a birthing hospital in the home. The organization was deeply concerned with the plight of unmarried mothers, who at the time were considered social outcasts with few options.

Sometime in 1914, the Women's Social Department was approached by some prominent citizens of Covington about the possibility of converting the mansion into a Protestant hospital for the city. The idea

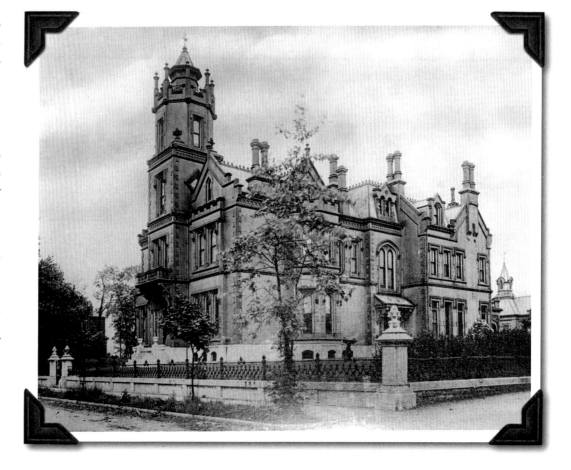

16 *Encyclopedia of Northern Kentucky*, p. 826; see also Norman H. Murdoch, *A Centennial History: The Salvation Army in Cincinnati, 1885–1985* (Cincinnati, Ohio: The Salvation Army Cincinnati, 1985).

was met with enthusiasm by the members of the Salvation Army, who appointed May Morgan, a major in the church, to head the new hospital.[17] The new hospital was to be named the William

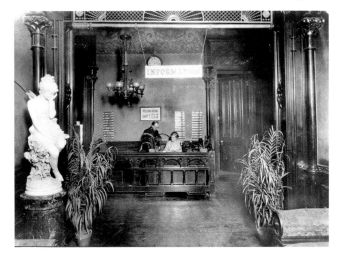 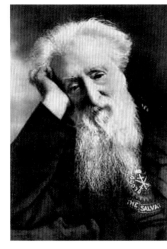

Lobby of Booth Hospital in the old Shinkle Mansion on E. 2nd St. From: St. Elizabeth Healthcare.

Right: William Booth, founder of the Salvation Army. From: Salvation Army website.

Opposite left: Nurses in yard of the old Shinkle Mansion, 1920s. From: St. Elizabeth Healthcare.

Opposite right: Booth Hospital School of Nursing, 3rd and Garrard Sts., Covington. From: photo by Raymond E. Hadorn, in the collection of Paul A. Tenkotte, Ph.D.

Booth Memorial Hospital, after the founder of the Salvation Army. In the spirit of the Salvation Army, the new hospital would "not patronize one class of people, but reach out to all."[18] The supporters in Covington immediately went to work to raise $100,000 to convert the building into a state-of-the-art hospital, although the hospital had already begun its development prior to the raising of the funds.

On May 26, 1915, the campaign for the hospital had nearly reached its goal. The *Kentucky Post* announced the names of some of the major contributors to the fund drive including an anonymous donor who gave $10,000. Smaller donors

included the Masons of Covington, Trinity Methodist Church, an African-American Church on Ninth Street and several ladies societies. Earlier that week, the Salvation Army sponsored a parade through Covington that drew 35,000 spectators and featured automobiles and the Salvation Army Band.[19] The highlight of the year was the arrival of Commander Evangeline Booth, daughter of William Booth, who spoke at the First Presbyterian Church in Covington. The British commander had been on a tour of America, speaking at various churches, and took the opportunity to see the new hospital in early February 1915. At the occasion of Evangeline Booth's speech about the life of her father, the board took the opportunity to showcase to the public its plans for improvements. These plans were met with high praise from Commander Booth, adding to the excitement of the evening.[20]

When it first opened, Booth Hospital had two major features which would become part of the hospital's hallmarks. The first was a large and modern maternity department, which was one of the first parts of the hospital to be modernized. It is possible that it was the success of the Booth Hospital maternity ward that persuaded the doctors at St. Elizabeth Hospital to request the creation of a maternity ward from the Diocese of Covington a few years later. A second important feature of the new hospital was its nursing school, which graduated its first class of registered nurses in December 1915. This initial nurs-

17 *Kentucky Post*, November 13, 1914, p. 1.

18 *Kentucky Post*, November 13, 1914, p. 1.

19 *Kentucky Post*, May 24, 1915, p. 1.

20 *Kentucky Post*, February 3, 1915, p. 4.

ing class numbered 15, which was a larger class than other nursing schools in the area at the time. The rigorous training and the camaraderie felt by nurses at Booth formed a unique atmosphere of pride and professionalism that few other hospitals could match. Even today, years after the closing of

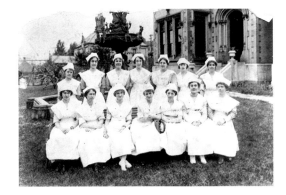

Booth Hospital, the former nurses of Booth still carry on with the same spirit and pride that were trademarks of their organization.

During the early 1920s, a flu epidemic struck Northern Kentucky. Hospitals in the area were taxed beyond their capacity. Booth set aside two wards for influenza patients and was forced to turn many away. The most important drain on the hospital's resources was the maternity ward and the surgery cases. These important functions could not be limited or restricted without potential loss of life, but less severe cases could be postponed.[21] It became clear to the leadership of Booth that the hospital

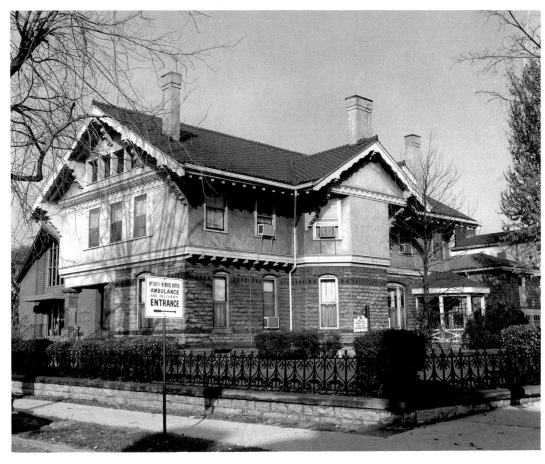

needed to expand. On June 12, 1920, the *Kentucky Post* reported that the hospital would raise enough money to build a new wing on the hospital, giving it enough capacity to meet its needs into the future.[22]

Unfortunately, the timing of the campaign was not good. A month later, the leadership of the Booth drive to raise $250,000

decided to postpone the campaign. One of the reasons cited was the fact that the hot summer weather had driven most of the community's leaders out of town to escape the heat, leaving the town short of those asking for donations and those giving donations. Another problem cited was the failure of the prior season's tobacco crop, which left many wealthy farmers in the area short of cash, thus limiting their ability

---

21 *Kentucky Post*, June 1, 1920, p. 1.

22 *Kentucky Post*, June 12, 1920, p. 1.

to donate. It was decided by the leadership that the campaign for Booth's new wing would be postponed until the fall.[23]

Booth Hospital's ongoing space problem and ongoing money challenges were oddly linked. In July 1920, the hospital reported that 40 percent of the patients it treated on a yearly basis were charity cases.[24] This meant that nearly half the people using the hospital made little or no payment for the services they received, including maternity and surgery services. In 1920 nearly 100 babies were born at Booth, and surgeries for the month of June that year numbered 137.[25]

In addition to the high number of charity cases and the continual need to raise money for expansion, Booth Hospital had an additional need. Because of the continued growth of the organization and the fact that a number of nurses left to aid the war effort in World War I, Booth suffered from a nursing shortage. In an attempt to end this shortfall, it was decided to expand and enhance the nurses' training program at the hospital. In December 1920, Booth acquired the former W.W. Brown Mansion on Garrard Street to be used as a home for students while they attended the nursing school. The purchase of the large home was made possible by a generous gift of $10,000

WM. BOOTH MEMORIAL HOSPITAL

Rates effective December 1, 1948

***

Six bed Wards	....	$6.50 per day
Four bed Wards	....	7.00 per day
Two bed rooms	....	8.25 per day
Private rooms	....	9.50 and
		11.00 per day

Maternity Rates

Room rates same as above. There is an additional charge of $22.50 for routine delivery service, $1.25 per day for the care of the baby and a $2.00 charge for circumcision.

Tonsillectomy Rates

Room rates same as above. There will be a flat charge of $10.00 for operating room and routine laboratory fees. There will be an extra charge for medications.

Room rates, Booth Hospital, 1948.
From: St. Elizabeth Healthcare.

by John A. Simpson in honor of his mother. Simpson was a wealthy merchant who had made his fortune in the dry goods business. His mother, Amelia, had been a school teacher who had supported the family after the death of her husband in the 1850s.[26] The new home was given the name Amelia Winston Simpson Rest.

Booth Hospital's campaign to raise money for a new wing and to pay off old debts got an unexpected boost in the spring of 1921. Jeff Davis, the self proclaimed "King of the Hobos," volunteered to help raise money for the hospital, saying that he wanted to help the folks of the "old army" because of their work among the poor. Davis, a writer, advocate, poet and shameless self-promoter, had gathered quite a following in the 1920s with his tales of life on the road. Americans at the time were in love with tales of the road and the romance of the vagabond life. Davis' image of the American hobo was that of a good man down on his luck riding the rails for more opportunity or for a chance at adventure. "The King of the Hobos" offer to help the Booth fund-raising campaign added a certain level of lightheartedness and underlined the importance of the hospital to the working poor. Throughout the 1920s, Booth continued to announce a number of expansion projects and fund-raising campaigns. Money raised was used to buy new equipment, add a fourth floor onto the building and build additions to the hospital grounds. Soon all that remained of the original Shinkle mansion were the four stone fence pillars located on a corner of the hospital lot.

The culmination of all the fundraising and expansion of the hospital was the opening of a new Booth Hospital in October 1926. The new building boasted nearly

23 Kentucky Post, July 17, 1920, p. 1.

24 Kentucky Post, July 7, 1920, p. 1.

25 Kentucky Post, July 7, 1920, p. 1.

26 United States census for the city of Covington, 1850 and 1860.

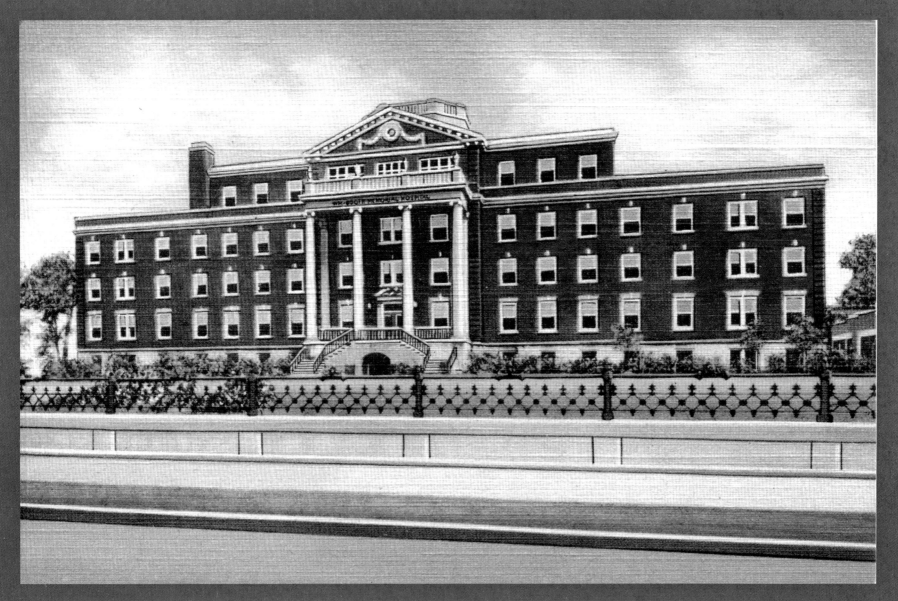

Postcard view of Booth Hospital, circa 1926. From: Paul A. Tenkotte, Ph.D.

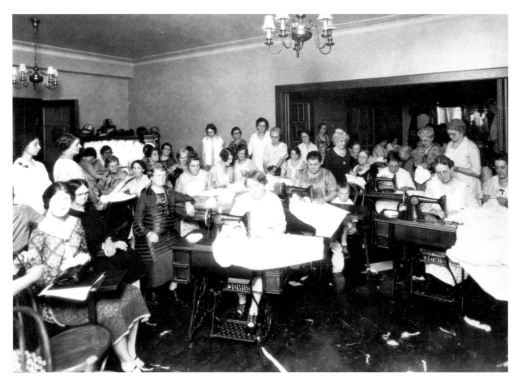

Volunteers sewing for Booth Hospital, 1926. From: St. Elizabeth Healthcare.

Opposite: Flood of 1937, Booth Hospital. From: St. Elizabeth Healthcare.

100 beds, two surgery rooms, an emergency room, cold water pumped directly from the city ice plant and a special clock in the maternity ward used for accurately recording the birth of each new baby born in the ward.[27]

Just as the new Booth Hospital was beginning to hit its stride, the nation was struck by the Great Depression. The number of charity cases, which had been high before, grew to record levels. In 1932, the hospital estimated that its annual operating deficit was $30,000, largely because of the services the hospital performed for those who

could not pay.[28] The first attempt to save money was the closing of the nursing school, announced in June 1932. The Great Depression had caused a surplus of nurses on the market due to layoffs and the fact that money-strapped hospitals everywhere were no longer hiring. Unfortunately, the closing of the nursing school was not enough. In August, Florence Turkington, superintendent of Booth Hospital, announced that the hospital would close its doors until economic factors improved. On September 1, 1932, the hospital discharged its last patient.[29]

True to the promise made at the closing of the hospital, Booth reopened five years later in January 1937, just in time for the worst natural disaster in Northern Kentucky's history. On that day, rains in the Cincinnati area added water to an Ohio River already near flood stage. It continued to rain on and off for the next 10 days forcing the river to rise to 79.99 feet, 27 feet above flood stage. Without the protection of a floodwall, water ran freely through the streets of Newport, Covington, Dayton and Ludlow. Water also ran freely though the basement of Booth Hospital causing considerable damage. During the flood, 50 people were forced from their homes and took up refuge in the hospital, despite its lack of heat and electricity.

In May 1937, the hospital kicked off a major campaign to pay for its flood damage, which amounted to $28,750. Five hundred volunteers were recruited and sent as far south as Florence

27 *The Kentucky Post*, August 13, 1926, p. 1, and May 5, 1927, p. 8.

28 *Kentucky Post*, September 1, 1932, p. 1.

29 *Kentucky Post*, September 1, 1932.

to seek aid. Each volunteer was asked to find and solicit 10 prospects for donations.[30] Solicitation for money, when so many Northern Kentuckians had lost so much, must have been difficult, but

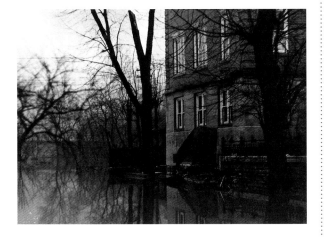

the community rose to the occasion. Fraternal organizations, churches, civic clubs and many individuals gave money for the repair of Booth. Soon the newly reopened hospital was at full capacity once again.

The hospital's return to patient care in Northern Kentucky could not have been better timed. In 1940, the *Kentucky Post* reported that Booth was continuing to see record growth. In 1939 alone, the hospital had witnessed nearly a 25 percent increase in service to the community in just one year.[31] One of the largest growth areas for the hospital was its maternity ward. In 1939 the hospital recorded 299 births. In May 1940, the hospital dedicated a new nursery to meet the growing

30　*Kentucky Post*, May 7, 1937.

31　*Kentucky Post*, January 25, 1940.

"We Laugh and Cry Together"

Glenna Mills, Human Resources Specialist, Benefits & Compensation Division

If you didn't know better, a walk by Glenna Mills' office might make you think she's always on the telephone with her family, what with the way she always seems to be saying "I love you too." At least that's what one new supervisor thought. But when she asked Glenna to whom she was talking, the supervisor learned it was just another St. Elizabeth associate that Glenna had helped complete important paperwork.

Helping people that she can both laugh and cry with has become a life's work for Glenna Mills. Now in her 41st year as an associate, Glenna worked the first three years at Speers Hospital in Dayton, Kentucky. At that time Speers was a 98-bed facility and Glenna started in the nutrition department. Meals then were nothing like they are now. Back then, she recalls, "unless you had a special dietary need, you ate what was put in front of you." Seeking and finding opportunities to learn new skills, Glenna also worked in purchasing, the business office and in medical records. When Speers closed, she joined the St. Elizabeth "family" and now helps people with their benefits or their retirement paperwork.

How many people today can remember record keeping before computers? Glenna can. She remembers that getting the first computer in Human Resources was "scary and amazing. ... You could put all this information in a small box and print it out three months later." The first computer, a Wang, which they all called "The Wang," had a small black screen with green letters. The computer and the printer took up an entire room.

Although it makes sense that someone in Human Resources would have memories that focus on "people," how Glenna Mills talks about St. Elizabeth and its people reveals something special. In Glenna's eyes, "everyone [she's known] is memorable ... people are Number 1 ... you and your family," at St. Elizabeth. Working in a faith-based institution also means a lot to Glenna, because sometimes, even in her work, she hears stories of suffering and "all you can offer them is prayer." That is not only allowed but supported at St. Elizabeth.

What keeps so many associates working for St. Elizabeth for decades? According to Glenna it comes down to just a few things. First, in her opinion, "St. Elizabeth wants to give us the best it can give us"—whether it's medical care for patients or a great place to work for the associates. Second, and most important, is the love and concern St. Elizabeth associates show for each other—be it prayers and well wishes when you or a family member is sick, or like Glenna's grandson, serving his country overseas, or if there's a birthday or a new baby to celebrate. That there's no real line between your personal family, your St. Elizabeth family and the larger family that is Northern Kentucky is also a reason why Glenna proudly concludes "St. Elizabeth is the top medical place to go."

Right: Groundbreaking for Booth Hospital, Florence, 1977. From: St. Elizabeth Healthcare.

Below left: Cafeteria, Booth Hospital, Covington, circa 1950s. Col. Wood, hospital administrator, is standing at the far left of the line. About halfway down the line is Virginia Clare, RN, who later became assistant director of nursing at St. Elizabeth Hospital. From: St. Elizabeth Healthcare.

Below right: Booth Hospital, Florence, opening year 1979. From: Kenton County Public Library, Covington.

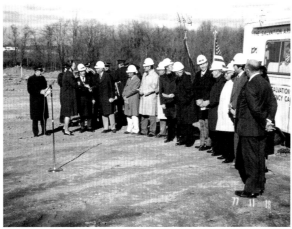

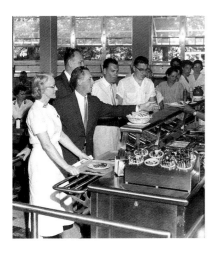

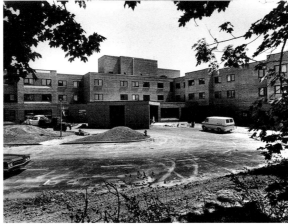

capacity of 60 additional beds. The *Kentucky Post* reported that the hospital was operating at over 90 percent capacity, with 137 beds occupied out of a total of 147.[32] The same day that the hospital announced its plan for more beds, the newspaper reported that the mayor of Covington applied to the United States Housing Authority for a permit to build 100 new homes to help alleviate an acute housing shortage. The city was growing by leaps and bounds, and Booth Hospital was attempting to keep up with the growing demand.

Ironically, the growth that led to the building of Booth Hospital and to its many improvements and additions would eventually lead to the closing of the hospital. Rather than the lack of adequate funding or the inability to keep up-to-date with changing medical practices, changing demographics brought about the end of Booth Hospital in Covington. A population that was moving south away from the city forced the medical community to think about moving to where their patients lived. The building off of the I-71/I-75 interstate west of the city helped facilitate this conversation. In 1979, Booth Hospital opened a new state-of-the-art hospital in Florence, Kentucky. In doing so, the Salvation Army closed Booth Hospital in Covington after 65 years of service to the community. Ten years later, Booth Hospital in Florence was sold to St. Luke Hospital and became St. Luke Hospital West. After 75 years, the Salvation Army was no longer in the hospital business in Northern Kentucky.[33]

demand. The room was funded by the hospital's Women's Auxiliary, an organization which had become the hospital's largest supporter. The Booth Memorial Hospital Women's Auxiliary became the envy of hospitals everywhere for its ability to move projects forward.

On December 1, 1945, Booth Hospital announced that it was planning the construction of an additional wing. The new wing would have the

---

32 *Kentucky Post*, December 1, 1945.

33 *Encyclopedia of Northern Kentucky*, p. 105.

St. Luke Hospital

It is safe to say that St. Elizabeth Healthcare is a better healthcare network because of St. Luke Hospital. Like two superstar athletes who compete against each other time and time again, the competition made both stronger. Fortunately for the people of Northern Kentucky, the competition between these two heavyweights of healthcare paid a dividend in the form of the best healthcare in the region.

The story of St. Luke Hospital began in 1947, when seven physicians came together to discuss the need for a new hospital in Campbell County. They sought a hospital that was more centrally located and easily accessible to a population moving south from the river. A 1948 study of Campbell County showed that the county had less than one-third of the hospital beds needed for its population of 80,000 people.[34]

It was agreed that a hospital needed to be built and that money needed to be raised. The first step was to pass a bond issue allowing the county the $1 million needed to start the project. The idea of a new hospital for the county was an easy sell to the voters of Campbell County, who passed the bond measure by a margin of 86 percent.[35] This overwhelming support bolstered the work of the new hospital board, which eagerly

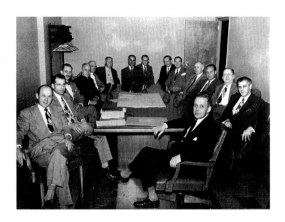

First Board of Trustees of St. Luke Hospital, 1954. From left and clockwise: Stanley C. Moebus; Paul R. Snyder; George F. Roth (architect of the hospital); Rev. Carl J. Merkle; Jacob Swope; Frank Sweigart; Michael A. Furio; Wesley Bowen (advisor); Rev. J. Paul Goebel; August H. Eilerman; Luther Bach, M.D. (advisor); Ervin G. Heiselman, M.D. (vice president); Oscar W. Frickman, M.D.; Mior Rifkin; Daniel D. Schwartz (president). From: St. Elizabeth Healthcare.

Below: Aerial view of St. Luke Hospital, Ft. Thomas. From: St. Elizabeth Healthcare.

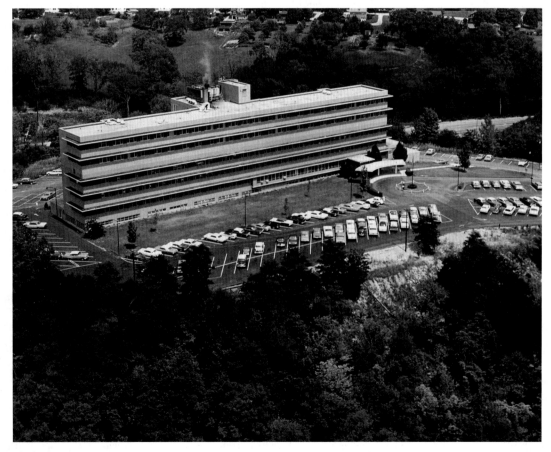

---

34 *The St. Luke Hospitals: 45 Years*, p. 1.

35 *The St. Luke Hospitals: 45 Years*, p. 1.

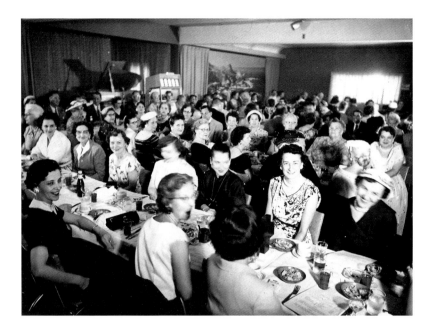

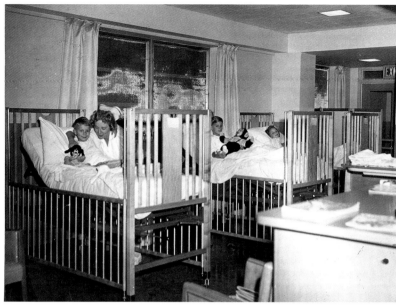

....

Cheery Cherry Pink Party was a fundraising event by ladies of a volunteer auxiliary of the hospital, circa 1960s. From: St. Elizabeth Healthcare.

Right: St. Luke Pediatric Tonsilarium, 1954. From: St. Elizabeth Healthcare.

Opposite: St. Luke Christmas babies, circa 1960s. From: St. Elizabeth Healthcare.

began working on the project. One of the first tasks was the selection of a name for the new hospital. The name chosen was St. Luke, after the writer of the third gospel of Jesus, who was reported to be a physician. A second task was to find a location that was easily accessible to all parts of the county. In all, 14 possible sites for the new hospital were considered. Finally, a section of land partially in Fort Thomas and partially in Newport seemed ideal and was secured for the new hospital.[36]

After some funding difficulties, caused in part by the Korean War, construction began in June 1952 on the $2.5 million St. Luke Hospital. Work was completed in two years, and the hospital was dedicated on July 4, 1954. Ironically, the

first patient arrived 10 days before the hospital officially opened, when a woman at the dedication ceremony became ill and needed to be treated at the emergency room.[37] The hospital's first administrator was R. Arthur Carvolth. Other important individuals who shaped the new hospital included Daniel Schwartz, who helped spearhead the bond issue, and Dr. Ervin G. Heiselman, who led the doctors' committee that first discussed the concept of a new hospital.

The new St. Luke Hospital boasted six operating rooms, a fully equipped maternity ward, and enough beds for 128 patients, more than doubling the bed capacity of Campbell County's other hospital, Speers Memorial. On the day after the official opening of St. Luke, the hospital ad-

36 *Kentucky Post,* April 6, 1949, p. 1.

37 *The St. Luke Hospitals: 45 Years,* p. 4.

mitted 11 patients, including two women who increased the number of patients to 13 by giving birth. The first official patient, not counting the woman who became ill at the dedication ceremony, was Mrs. Edward Shulte, who gave birth to a son, Clifford Luke Shulte, born July 14, 1954.[38]

The farsightedness of the hospital's founders was evident in how quickly the hospital became a major institution for the region. By 1957, it became clear that the hospital needed to grow. Another bond issue was passed by voters and in 1963 two new floors were added to the hospital, bringing the total bed capacity to 201.[39] Even this expansion was not enough. By the early 1970s the hospital was operating at 98 percent of capacity. In 1975, a south wing was added to the hospital, once again expanding the hospital's patient bed space, this time to 290.[40]

Almost from the beginning, St. Luke became a leader in healthcare for the region. In 1958 staff of the hospital implanted the first patient myocardial pacemaker in Northern Kentucky. This procedure for the heart was the first of many innovations related to heart health brought to the area by St. Luke. In 1970, the hospital opened the first coronary care unit in Northern Kentucky, saving the lives of many heart pa-

tients. Other firsts and innovations brought to the area by the hospital included chemotherapy treatments for cancer patients in 1975, the introduction of helicopter emergency medical service in 1978, and the first CT medical imaging scanner in 1980.

Also in 1980, St. Luke Hospital purchased the former Pendleton County Hospital in order to expand both inpatient and outpatient services for those trying to overcome substance abuse. The Pendleton

County Hospital, located in Falmouth Kentucky, had opened in 1966, largely due to the dedication of Dr. William Townsend and Dr. Robert McKenny. The original 28-bed hospital, providing emergency, surgical, infant delivery, and other services, had closed its doors in 1980. In 1982 St. Luke opened the Alcohol and Drug Treatment Center there, in conjunction with Careunit Inc. The facility was the first of its kind in Northern Kentucky. Even as recently as

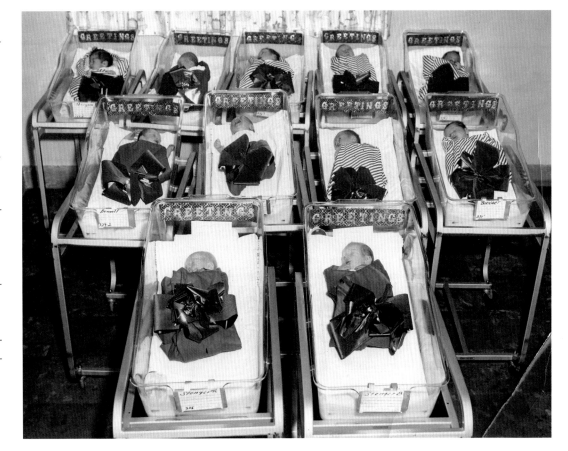

---

38 *The St. Luke Hospitals: 45 Years,* p. 4.

39 *The St. Luke Hospitals: 45 Years,* p. 5.

40 *The St. Luke Hospitals: 45 Years,* p. 6.

"Going into Missionary Medicine"

Cardio-Thoracic Surgeon Dr. George Hall

No one in Dr. George Hall's family had been in the medical profession; he even started college with the intent of becoming an accountant. So how did the Arkansas native from a family of farmers and teachers discover that he was meant to be a surgeon? After exploring the classes his pre-med friends were taking and realizing that he "just liked the subject matter better," Hall changed direction. Once on the path to becoming a doctor, Hall found that the decision to be a surgeon was the result of everything all falling together. Hall chose the University of Cincinnati for internship and residency because of its national reputation and because it was close enough that he could drive home within a day.

The 1970s proved to be an auspicious time to be a young doctor in the Greater Cincinnati area. "A lot of doctors were getting older and making room for younger" doctors—especially in Northern Kentucky, he recalls. But, there was still something about crossing the river that spurred comments. Running into an anesthesiologist in a grocery store, Hall remembers the native of Ft. Mitchell teasing him: "So I hear you're going into missionary medicine." That was her way of self-deprecatingly needling him about his decision to practice in Northern Kentucky. But Hall was not alone; several fellow residents from UC had preceded Hall in the move and thus when he "came over it was like old home week."

Dr. Hall first affiliated with St. Luke Hospital, an institution started in the 1950s "by men of vision." After merging with Booth, St. Luke eventually joined the Ohio-based

Health Alliance, but that "wasn't a particularly good fit." After at least two attempts, the merger with St. Elizabeth was achieved, when "personalities meshed...the stars aligned...[and] a spirit of 'let's just get on with it' took over."

Hall stresses two reasons for the merger's success. First, Joseph Gross and John Dubis invested in St. Luke, buying new equipment and making it easier for the hospital to better serve its patients. Second, "no one lost their job" because of the merger.

Even as St. Elizabeth marks its 150th anniversary, the separate identities of the institutions it has absorbed are remembered. When asked what he would want remembered about St. Luke, Hall asserted emphatically "its esprit-de-corps," that it was a place with a "family, home-away-from-home spirit."

The dedication of associates like Dr. George Hall ensures the success of the "better together" motto. Hall even abandoned retirement in Florida to play his part. Now vice president for medical affairs, Hall leads a division that credentials 1,100-plus doctors and allied health professionals every two years. The division also oversees the assessment of quality and patient safety, and risk management.

From his vantage point, Hall predicts a bright future for St. Elizabeth, with "more" as the key word. Hall foresees "more services ... more outreach ... especially for underserved populations." In final reflection, Hall shares that he is just "so thankful for having the opportunity to take care of people." Like so many at St. Elizabeth, George Hall is perhaps a missionary in spirit, if not in fact, after all.

the 1980s and the 1990s, such facilities for the treatment of chemical addiction were often the stepchild of the medical profession. Although recognized as a disease by most doctors, chemical dependency carried a stigma of being an addiction that "decent people" would not get. In the opinion of many Americans, chemical dependency was associated with criminals, not with one's neighbors. As a result, the unit had difficulty raising necessary funds, as well as meeting the challenge of reaching those in the community who needed help the most.

Fortunately, thanks to changes in social attitudes, and the publicity elicited by the chemical dependency stories of many celebrities in the popular media, the stigma of substance abuse lessened. Starting in the new century, many insurance companies changed their policies to support recovery services for those addicted to drugs and other chemicals. When St. Elizabeth Hospital merged with St. Luke Hospital, Falmouth became St. Elizabeth Falmouth, continuing its fine service to those in need. Today, St. Elizabeth Falmouth is the only hospital-based chemical dependency program in Northern Kentucky.

The hallmark of St. Luke Hospital was always to meet the needs of today while preparing for those of tomorrow. One of the needs that the hospital had the good sense to plan for was the possibility of an area disaster. In 1977 the hospital established a MEDVAN program with a fully equipped field disaster team. In addition, the hospital drilled its nurses and doctors with mock disasters in order to prepare them for real emergencies. St. Luke's trauma team practiced for the

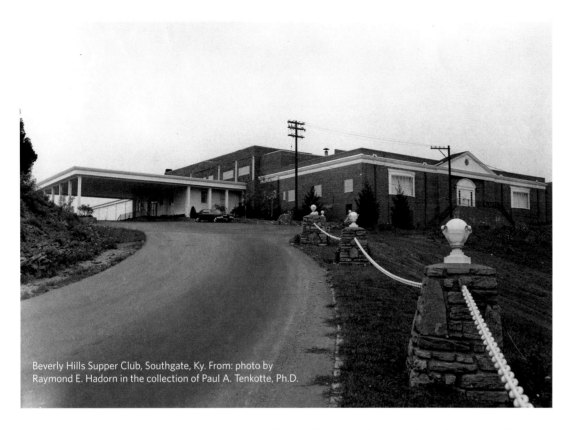
Beverly Hills Supper Club, Southgate, Ky. From: photo by Raymond E. Hadorn in the collection of Paul A. Tenkotte, Ph.D.

possibility of events with large numbers of casualties, including bus and plane crashes. The resulting practice brought about the development of a disaster plan which could be implemented at a moment's notice.

They did not have to wait too long for that moment. On May 28, 1977, fire broke out at the overcrowded Beverly Hills Supper Club in Southgate, Kentucky, near St. Luke. One of the people on the scene that night was St. Luke CEO John Hoyle, who had gone to the supper club for a night out. Hoyle's call to the emergency room at St.

Luke was short and to the point: "This is Hoyle. I am at the Beverly Hills. There is a very bad fire. Unknown number of casualties. Activate the disaster plan."[41] His words set in motion a crack disaster team, so well-trained that the hospital worked like a well-oiled machine. The hospital was ready when the first of the injured arrived and worked until the last victim was taken care of. Many doctors and nurses worked well

beyond the call of duty, working through multiple shifts.[42]

When the crisis was over, 165 people died as a result of the fire and 116 people were injured. Most of the injured were treated by St. Luke because it was the closest hospital to the fire. It is unknown how many lives were saved due to the preparedness of the hospital staff. One witness recalled that he had "never seen people work so well together, so efficiently."[43] It is safe to say that many people owe their lives to the efficiency of St. Luke's trauma team. The disaster plan worked so well that it became a model studied around the world by hospitals and government agencies wishing to develop their own disaster plans.

The 1980s were a time of incredible growth for St. Luke. The hospital not only added more beds and more patient rooms, but also centers for cancer treatment, substance abuse, a clinic for abused children, a birthing center, a diabetes center and a sleep disorder center. In 1989, St. Luke purchased the William Booth Memorial Hospital in Florence, Kentucky, renaming it St Luke Hospital West. The Fort Thomas hospital became known as St. Luke Hospital East. The purchase of Booth Hospital greatly expanded St. Luke's service area and offered more healthcare opportunities to the people of Northern Kentucky.

---

41 *The St. Luke Hospitals: 45 Years*, p. 7.

42 *The St. Luke Hospitals: 45 Years*, p. 7.

43 *The St. Luke Hospitals: 45 Years*, p. 7.

In 1995 St. Luke announced that it was joining the Health Alliance of Greater Cincinnati, combining resources with several other hospitals on the north side of the Ohio River. The alliance allowed the hospitals to pool their resources and offer a wider variety of healthcare options to the

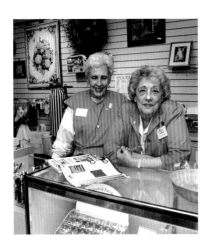

St. Luke Gift Shop, circa 1980s.
From: St. Elizabeth Healthcare.

Right: Ceremony commemorating the purchase of Booth Hospital by St. Luke Hospital, 1989. At the podium is Col. Paul Seiler. To his left seated is James White. From: St. Elizabeth Healthcare.

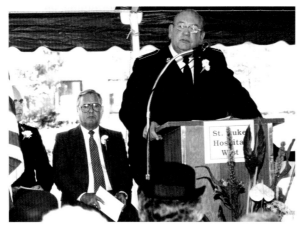

people of the region. The whole idea behind the alliance was to provide cost-savings by sharing the cost of some functions, such as laboratory and pharmaceutical work.

St. Luke's marriage to the Alliance was not a happy one. The challenge for the alliance was the monumental task of coordinating the coalition of hospitals and healthcare providers, each retaining its own leadership.[44] St. Luke, an organization that prided itself with forward-thinking people who moved quickly with the changing healthcare

landscape, often found the cumbersomeness of the alliance restrictive. In addition, the alliance's leadership was accused of directing business to preferred hospitals in exchange for kickbacks, thus leaving some hospitals and their medical staff underutilized. In May 2010, the alliance and Christ Hospital agreed to pay $108 million to settle federal lawsuits over illegal kickbacks for giving preference to some hospitals in the alliance over others.[45]

The people of St. Luke Hospital had always strived to bring the best in healthcare innovations to the people of Northern Kentucky. To many, the Health Alliance of Greater Cincinnati had become an obstacle that made fulfilling that mission more difficult. In 2006 St. Luke Hospitals and St. Elizabeth Hospital began to discuss the possibility of a merger. The partnership would allow St. Luke to dissolve its role in the partnership with the alliance, while allowing the hospital system to rededicate itself to the care of the Northern Kentucky community. The strengths of the two healthcare superstars complemented each other extremely well, and that was summed up by two very simple words: "Better Together."

The one major concern expressed by the leadership of both organizations was how the merger would affect the employees of each. After all, both institutions agreed, the one irreplaceable resource that they both shared was the dedicated, talented and motivated staff that made up the

44 "Cincinnati's Health Alliance Dissolves," *www.darkdaily.com* (Clinical Laboratory and Pathology New and Trends), accessed on January 28, 2011.

45 "Health Alliance of Greater Cincinnati, Christ Hospital Pay 108m to Settle Federal Kickback Accusations," *Becker's ASCReview: Practical Business, Legal and Clinical Guidance for Ambulatory Surgery Centers,* www.beckersasc.com, accessed on January, 28, 2011.

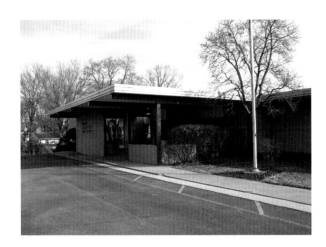

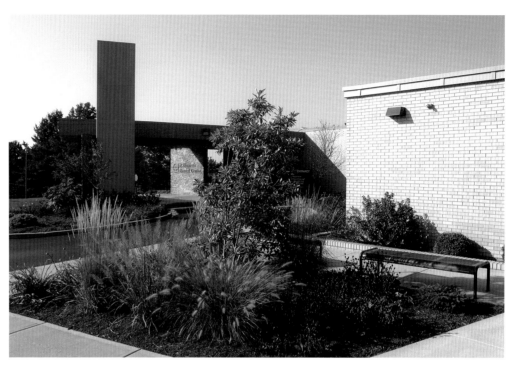

two healthcare families. It was agreed early in the merger conversations that any current employee who wanted to remain with the new organization would be allowed to stay. If the job that he or she had held previously was not needed, then the new St. Elizabeth Healthcare would give the employee the opportunity and support to gain new skills and find a new position within the system. This foresighted and generous act, at a time when most companies prided themselves on cutting their bottom line at the expense of loyal employees, is a testimony of how much the leadership recognized the value of its human assets.

The marriage of St. Luke and St. Elizabeth healthcare systems brings the history of healthcare in Northern Kentucky full circle. The area's first hospital, St. Elizabeth, opened in 1861 with the simple concept of helping Northern Kentuckians in need. That same spirit also motivated farsighted and caring people to open Speers, Booth, and St. Luke, continuing a legacy of fine healthcare for all people.

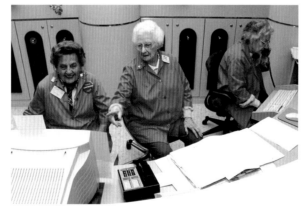

Top left: St. Elizabeth Falmouth, located in Falmouth, KY is an alcohol and drug treatment facility. Opened in 1981, Falmouth celebrated its 30th anniversary in 2011.

Above: St. Elizabeth Grant, located in Williamstown, KY. Originally opened in 1964 as Grant County Hospital, it became a part of St. Elizabeth in 1993.

Left: Volunteers, Information Desk, St. Luke Hospital, circa 1990s. From: St. Elizabeth Healthcare.

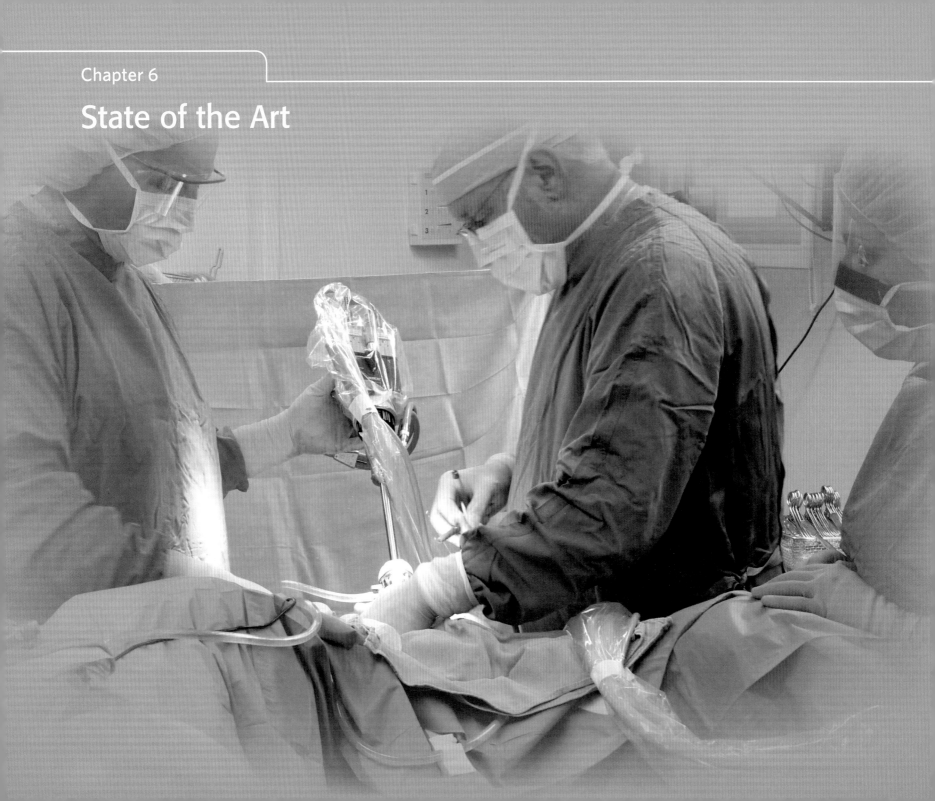

Chapter 6

State of the Art

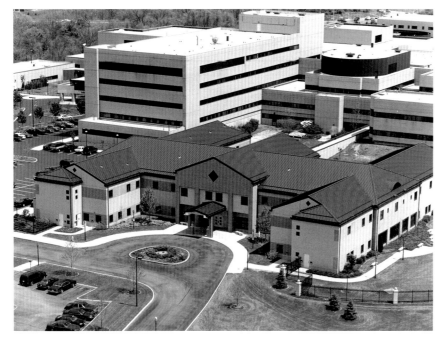

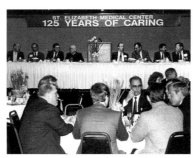

Aerial view of new Behavioral Health Center, 1997. From: St. Elizabeth Healthcare.

Left: St. Elizabeth 125th anniversary banquet, January 1987. From: St. Elizabeth Heathcare.

Previous page: Surgery using the new daVinci robot, St. Elizabeth, Edgewood, 2009. From: St. Elizabeth Healthcare.

One hundred fifty years ago, Northern Kentucky's only hospital, St. Elizabeth, had one building, ten beds, four nuns who served as nurses, and a budget made up almost entirely of what could be begged for, donated or picked up off the ground. There were fewer than five doctors who serviced the hospital when it first opened. Patients who came to the hospital were Protestant, Catholic, Jewish and even agnostic. They were black, white, slave, free, native born and immigrants. They were poor and hard-working, some having worked so hard that their bodies were worn out and there was no more work within them, leaving them with no place else to go. Some were hours old, some many years old, but they all needed what St. Elizabeth had to offer: a safe place to die or a chance to live.

The simple mission of Northern Kentucky's first hospital was to provide for the healthcare needs of the community regardless of race or creed. If the founders of the institution had a vision, it may simply have been to "serve others." They did what was needed for so many: finding solutions, embracing adversity and respecting all life. The struggle made them family. Their guidance was the Catholic Church, which offered support and direction. It stood as a rock when the challenges seemed to be so overwhelming. Over time, this small beacon of light and caring that refused to surrender to the darkness of ignorance, prejudice, poverty and tremendous community needs became such a part of the community that they seemed inseparable.

Now jump ahead 150 years. St. Elizabeth Healthcare has 6 hospitals, 50 primary care offices, 3 free-standing imaging center buildings, more than 1,000 beds and 6,300 direct employees with nearly 1,000 other associated employees. It has more than 1,200 physicians with admitting privileges and an annual budget of hundreds of mil-

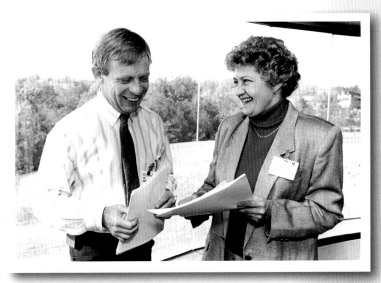

St. Elizabeth Vision Campaign Chairs, Tim McDermott and Joyce Julien, 1997. From: St. Elizabeth Healthcare.

lions of dollars. The hospitals and doctors of St. Elizabeth Healthcare serve people of all faiths, races and backgrounds. As it was 150 years ago, St. Elizabeth is the only hospital in Northern Kentucky. The nuns are no longer nurses, nor do they run the

"The Mayor of St. Elizabeth": Tim McDermott

Born at St. Elizabeth to a mother who trained in the St. Elizabeth nursing school and went on to work in the emergency room, Tim McDermott personifies the many St. Elizabeth associates whose families have multiple and generational connections to the institution. Hired in 1968 when "the good nuns" were still in charge, McDermott reflects back on more than 40 years of service at St. Elizabeth with pride and love. Once during an orientation tour, after noting how many associates spoke to Tim by name and vice versa, one gentleman remarked, "Who are you—the mayor of St. Elizabeth?"

Tim McDermott is a living connection to St. Elizabeth traditions, past, present and future. With authority he notes, "St. Elizabeth anniversaries have always been a celebration of the St. Elizabeth family." Remembering the North Unit annual festival, Tim admits that he doesn't know if the hospital made any money, but for the kids "with horse rides, dime bingo, you name it," the event was a big hit. Like most St. Elizabeth associates, Tim stresses how "good the hospital has been to me." Starting as a surgical orderly just out of the Navy, Tim went to school to become a nurse and worked his way up to become nurse manager of the North Unit surgery. One of Tim's proudest moments came when the South Unit opened and he came over to help teach labor and delivery nurses how to do C-sections. Another activity near to Tim's heart has been 16

years as co-director of employee fundraising for the Vision Campaign; notable achievements being the establishment of the Employee Crisis Line and Employee Fitness Center. Why does Tim feel so strongly about St. Elizabeth? He explains, "It doesn't make any difference if you're the president or in housekeeping—we appreciate your work."

Devotion imbues every story Tim tells, even the Sister Ascentia ghost story. Never a believer in ghosts, Tim's view changed one night at the North Unit. Heading toward a corner, Tim saw a nun and stopped short because he didn't want to run into her, which he didn't "because she was gone." According to his mother and other nurses he spoke with, Sister Ascentia appeared whenever someone on the floor was going to die—which happened the night Tim saw her. Asked why a nun would reappear in ghostly form, Tim and even retired Sisters of the Poor stated unequivocally that in life her mission was to care for the dying and that her appearances are proof that she remains devoted to helping others make that journey.

McDermott's memories illuminate the uplifting and loving spirit at the heart of St. Elizabeth. Recalling the ice storm of 1977, Tim notes with chagrin that the nurses and staff spent the night stranded at the hospital "with all the food in the world ... playing euchre" while their spouses "were stuck at home with the kids." From this lighthearted memory to St. Elizabeth's addition of hospice care, Tim's stories focus on the positive. Now caring for people through the entire "continuum of birth, life and death," St. Elizabeth through its hospice care helps its patients focus on the joys of their lives, even as death approaches. No wonder Tim McDermott says "we" when speaking of St. Elizabeth. He speaks not just for himself, but for generations.

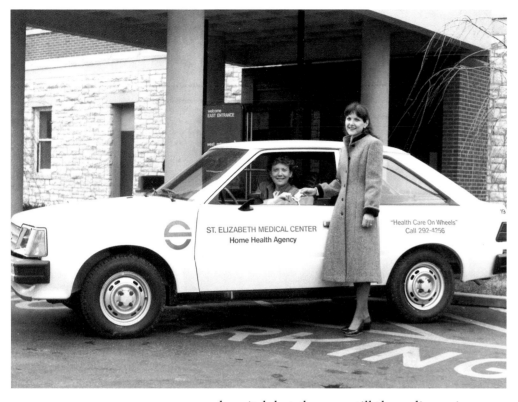

Pat Furnish, RN, seated in car, director of the St. Elizabeth Medical Center Home Health/Hospice department, receives keys from St. Elizabeth Auxiliary president Diane Abbing. By 1983, the year of this photo, the auxiliary had purchased 12 automobiles for the department's use in treating the sick of the Northern Kentucky community. From: St. Elizabeth Healthcare.

Right: St. Elizabeth North volunteer Mildred Canfield and a clown visit with a young patient, 1984. From: St. Elizabeth Healthcare.

countrymen, the Ohio River is not the barrier between communities it once was and hospitals are not institutions to be feared as many people once believed. We have changed a lot in 150 years and so has St. Elizabeth Healthcare.

Healthcare in America is a more than $2 trillion industry[1] that has regulations, standards and ratings in place. Its clinical employees must master the melding of two powerful and often conflicting forces—the compassionate care needs of patients and the ever-changing advances of science. Most importantly, it has a customer base that demands the best care it can get. The truly modern healthcare institution is judged by many standards, including ratings by agencies within the profession, employees, patients, community leaders and the community served.

St. Elizabeth Healthcare's awards and recognitions are a testimony to the legacy of excellence that hard work brings. St. Elizabeth has been in the top 5 percent in the nation for the past five

hospital, but they are still there dispensing comfort and peace as their fellow sisters did years before. One may ask, does the current incarnation of St. Elizabeth Hospital still care for the poor? The answer would be "yes." In 2009, St. Elizabeth Healthcare provided $100 million in community benefits and uncompensated care. Of that amount, $63 million went to community care such as health fairs, free screenings and other community education events. The remaining $37 million went to help those who could not pay for medical services.

But things are different now. America is not the same place. We are not at war with our fellow

1 U.S. Healthcare costs, *www.KaiserEDU.org* educational website for the Kaiser Foundation, accessed on January 31, 2011.

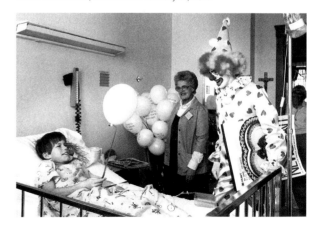

"The Cap Doesn't Make the Nurse"

Jana McElroy, Regional Diabetes Center

Many, if not most nurses of Jana McElroy's generation, had an aunt who was also a nurse, but Jana remembers a summer reading list book having the deciding influence on the course of her life. The book told the story of Father Damien, who cared for the lepers of Hawaii. His selfless devotion to caring for those whom others had abandoned inspired Jana even though television shows could make her squeamish. Jana's sensitivity inspired skepticism in her father; when he was told that she wanted to be a nurse, he proclaimed that he "wouldn't give two bucks" that she would make it. But she did.

As a member of the last class of the St.Elizabeth nursing school, Jana needed every ounce of her courage. Jana and her classmates (who included Ruth Henthorn) endured what she described as "a baptism by fire"—there were three plane crashes in the three years of their training. Still able to recall the smell of the burned, fuel-soaked flesh of the victims, Jana says, makes her think of what her father, who was at Pearl Harbor, and her aunt, who was a World War II Navy nurse, must have experienced. One of the positive memories from those horrible events Jana recalls is the story of Toni Ketchall, a pretty young stewardess and crash survivor who fought to keep a leg and not only "came back to us" for all of her surgeries, but also attended the graduation of the student nurses who helped care for her. In Jana's eyes, this was a real testament to the care she received.

Among the members of class dubbed "the Wave Makers," Jana served in behavioral health, the ICU and nurses' training before finding her niche in diabetes education. What's the connection between making waves and diabetes education? Empowerment! First, Jana says that being

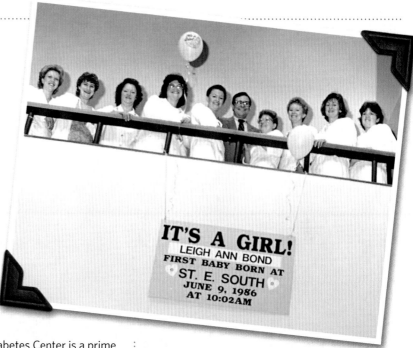

First baby born at St. Elizabeth South was Leigh Ann Bond, June 9, 1986. From: St. Elizabeth Healthcare.

IT'S A GIRL!
LEIGH ANN BOND
FIRST BABY BORN AT
ST. E. SOUTH
JUNE 9, 1986
AT 10:02AM

one of the Wave Makers meant that she and her generation spoke up more. Because they were encouraged to do so they feel a great sense of accomplishment in the advances, particularly in patient care, that have been a hallmark of St. Elizabeth through the years. And when it comes to empowerment through education, St. Elizabeth's Regional Diabetes Center is a prime example of the 21st century innovations that St. Elizabeth is gaining a reputation for. From the humble beginnings 30 years ago, when doctors would submit requests to have a nurse show a patient how to give themselves insulin injections, through the establishment in 1988 of a formal diabetes education program (with two educators and a dietician), and now with a state-of the art facility that streamlines diagnostic, preventive, educational, and ancillary services (think one-stop shopping for diabetes care), Jana McElroy has been proud to be a part of an initiative that focuses on empowering patients through education and support. The evolution and transformation of her role and of so many other St. Elizabeth associates is illuminated by this story she tells:

While she was still an ICU nurse, they had a young male patient who was comatose, but the doctors instructed the nurses to talk to him and encourage him even though he couldn't respond. Miraculously he pulled through and one day, while Jana and another nurse were helping him walk around the unit, they were stopped by someone who wanted to know why they (the nurses) didn't have on their caps. (They had taken them off because he was still hooked up to so much that they couldn't keep all that straight and keep their caps in place.) Without missing a beat, the young man looked the inquisitor up and down and said, "The cap doesn't make the nurse."

At St. Elizabeth the focus has always been on the patient and the community. That legacy just keeps growing.

"We're Still Here and Getting Better and Better"

John S. Dubis, St. Elizabeth Healthcare President and Chief Executive Officer

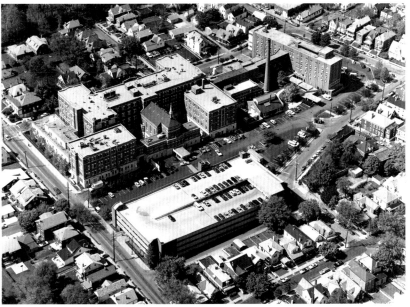

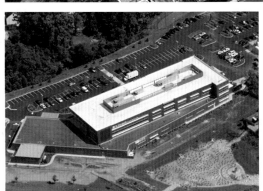

Aerial photo of the new St. Elizabeth Covington, 2009. From: St. Elizabeth Healthcare.

Top: Aerial view of St. Elizabeth North, 20th St., Covington, 1992. From: St. Elizabeth Healthcare.

When asked what he wanted the people of the future to know about St. Elizabeth, John S. Dubis, President and Chief Executive Officer, replied without hesitation, "We're still here and getting better and better." Although he wasn't seeking a job when approached by a friend about St. Elizabeth, Dubis found himself swayed after hearing about the organization's commitment to quality, clinical excellence and its record of compassionate care. Following a visit to Northern Kentucky, and convinced that these were hallmarks of St. Elizabeth's workplace culture, Dubis came to St. Elizabeth in 2008.

Following Joe Gross, during whose 25-year tenure at St. Elizabeth "developed ... into something really outstanding," Dubis declares that he is dedicated to seeing the organization continue on that path. Echoing his predecessor, Dubis points to three hallmarks of achievement that illuminate St. Elizabeth's prominence: named one of America's 50 Best Hospitals by HealthGrades for the fifth year in a row (2007–2011), named a 100 Top Hospital by Thomson Reuters six times including five years in a row (1998, 2007–2011),

and was the first hospital to achieve Magnet™ status for nursing care in 2006 and being re-designated again in 2010. Underscoring the last achievement, Dubis notes that "only three other hospitals in the country have concurrently earned these three prestigious honors."

How will St. Elizabeth maintain such momentum and remain "a premium center of excellence"? Dubis foresees focusing on providing care for more people through a seamless delivery system that is comprehensive, non-fragmented and state of the art. For example, in 2008, St. Elizabeth purchased an Aquilion ONE 320-slice CT Scanner that can create a 3-D diagnostic image of the human heart in a fraction of a second; when purchased it was one of 10 in use in the entire world. EPIC, the online, electronic patient records system used by the healthcare system, puts a patient's entire medical profile at the fingertips of his or her medical team. Consolidation of service sites, such as the creation of the Regional Diabetes Center, allows patients to go to one location to receive care for multiple issues like nutritional counseling, the treatment of diabetes and endocrine disorders and wound care. Finally, St. Elizabeth continues to expand its outreach and mobile care services. From the 900 employees of Aurora Casket served by a St. Elizabeth Physicians clinic in Dearborn County, Indiana, to the patrons of the Mobile Mammography Van and the CardioVascular Mobile Health Unit, the people of the Northern Kentucky-Greater Cincinnati region will continue to be cared for by an organization that Dubis firmly believes one day will rival nationally known medical centers like the Mayo Clinic.

years as rated by HealthGrades, a leading independent healthcare ratings company. It has been ranked as one of the nation's 100 Top Hospitals by Thomson Reuters, a leading source for information on technology and business recognized worldwide for its accuracy and diligence in business ratings. In addition, the hospital achieved Magnet™ Status by the American Nurses Credentialing Center of the American Nursing Association in 2006, and was re-designated in 2010. Only two other hospitals in the nation have received all three of these rankings at the same time.

While in 2007 *U.S. News and World Report* identified St. Elizabeth as one of America's top 50 hospitals for respiratory care and endocrinology, the organization has also received national or regional awards for many other areas of specialty including diabetes care, women's health, cardiac and stroke, gastrointestinal, orthopaedics, spine care and surgery, patient safety, emergency medicine and critical care.

In addition to these awards, St. Elizabeth Healthcare has consistently ranked as one of the Best Places to Work by the *Cincinnati Business Courier*, the Kentucky Chamber of Commerce and the employees of St. Elizabeth Healthcare. Because this award is voted on by employees, it speaks volumes about St. Elizabeth Healthcare as an organization. The employees, or associates as they are now called, often refer to St. Elizabeth as a family. Together they have

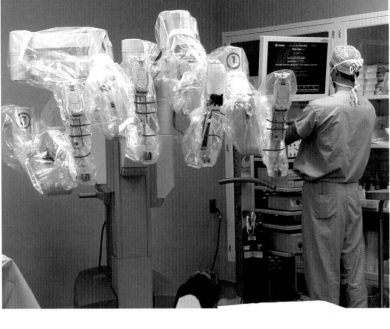

The daVinci robot used for precise surgery, 2009. From: St. Elizabeth Healthcare.

shared their personal triumphs and tragedies, helping to make the organization much more than a place to work. Not surprisingly, the feeling that St. Elizabeth is a family seems to have existed from its early founding 150 years ago.

One large piece of evidence of this family atmosphere is found in the St. Elizabeth Healthcare Foundation. The Foundation, like so many healthcare foundations around the country, raises money for special projects within the healthcare system. What is special about the Foundation at St. Elizabeth Healthcare is the commitment that employees of the hospital have shown to the Foundation and its projects.

Most institutions would feel blessed if they receive 50 percent participation from their employees in a fund-raising campaign, with many attaining only about 30 percent involvement. St. Elizabeth routinely has more than 80 percent participation. A possible reason for this astonishing level of

support is the fact that the associates at St. Elizabeth truly believe in the work of the institution and in helping the community. The St. Elizabeth Healthcare Foundation works every day with hundreds of individuals, organizations and businesses to raise the funds needed to give our community the best healthcare available. With a Foundation volunteer board and committee base of nearly 200 business and community leaders, the winners in all of this are the people we serve—the thriving population of Northern Kentucky and Greater Cincinnati.

Over the years, the Foundation's bi-annual "Vision" campaign has raised money for the purchase of a da Vinci surgical robot, a mobile health screening van and its latest

"Once a Nurse, Always a Nurse"

Beatrice Luella Jacobs Bradley,
oldest living St. Elizabeth Nursing School graduate

"Once a nurse, always a nurse," replied Sister Mary Anthony to Lu Bradley after she resisted the sister's offer to return to nursing after a 20-year absence. Galvanized by the sister's simple retort, Bradley returned to St. Elizabeth and served as a "Med-Surg" nurse from 1960 to 1978. Now the oldest living graduate from St. Elizabeth's nursing school, Bradley's memories range from the details of daily life of early 20th century student nurses, to how St. Elizabeth staff responded to challenges, to the dramatic transformations in patient care.

Like many nurses, Bradley was inspired to become a nurse by the example of female relatives, in her case, an aunt. A native of Ironton, Ohio, Bradley first looked into a program at Berea, but after learning that the student nurses had to wear black stockings, which was "for the birds," she selected the St. Elizabeth program.

Life as a student nurse was hard but also fun. Monday through Friday, six young women shared a room, rose at 6 a.m. for Mass and breakfast followed by classes and service on the wards. During the week, they had to be in by 9 p.m., but could stay out until 11 p.m. one night a week. Sharing clothes and arranging dates for each other, the student nurses enjoyed attending movies, plays and dances, not unlike other young people. In fact, according to Bradley, the change in the St. Elizabeth nursing cap from square to pointed tip was inspired by a movie—1934's *White Parade*, starring Loretta Young. Of her time as a student, Bradley asserts, "I loved every minute of it!"

Bradley's early memories of St. Elizabeth in the 1930s offer insight into a recurring theme in the St. Elizabeth story—"there's always a way," or resilience in the face of adversity. In the depths of the Great Depression, the nuns made soup in a big black kettle on the hospital grounds from vegetables provided by farmers. Bradley still remembers people standing in the soup line "four to five abreast."

When Bradley started her training, there was one bathroom per hall of patients. To bathe a patient, the nurses had to carry water in pails and use a basin for the washing. When doctors ordered ice chips for patients, the ice had to be crushed manually. Returning to nursing in 1960, Bradley discovered "night and day" type changes. A particular change Bradley noted was the passing of the days of "sterilizing everything" to giving shots with plastic syringes.

Looking back on all of her experiences, Bradley proudly proclaims, "I'd do the same old thing all over again, and I wouldn't trade my training or work for a million bucks."

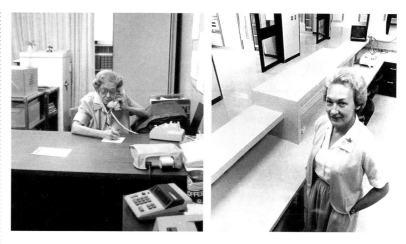

Left: Volunteer Loretta Gibson donated over 20,000 hours to St. Elizabeth, 1987. From: St. Elizabeth Healthcare.

Right: Rose Hook graduated from St. Elizabeth School of Nursing in 1953. She served as vice president of nursing at St. Elizabeth for 22 years. When she retired in 1996, she had served at St. Elizabeth Hospital for 43 years. From: Kenton County Public Library, Covington.

project, the most powerful X-ray imaging device on the planet, the Toshiba Aquilion One 320-Slice CT Scanner. It is easy to say that without the strong support of the community and the employees of St. Elizabeth Healthcare, the efforts of the Foundation would not be nearly as successful. This is a fact that is not lost on the Foundation and its supporters, who see the people of St. Elizabeth as being part of their strength.

Would Henrietta Cleveland, Sarah Worthington King Peter, Bishop Carrell, Frances Schervier and the first four German sisters who came to America to operate St. Elizabeth recognize their hospital in St. Elizabeth Healthcare today? Aside from the state-of-the-art technology and the overwhelming enormity of the size of the institution, the answer would be a resounding "yes!" The mission and the vision that shaped the hospital so many years ago are still very much alive and reflected in the people of St. Elizabeth and in the community it has so faithfully served for so long.

Index

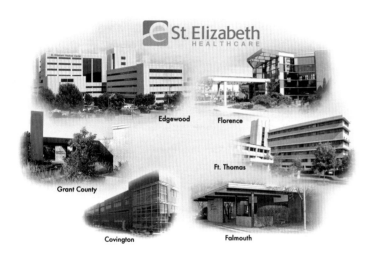

St. Elizabeth HEALTHCARE

Edgewood

Florence

Ft. Thomas

Grant County

Covington

Falmouth

About St. Elizabeth Healthcare Today

St. Elizabeth Healthcare has six hospitals in Covington, Edgewood, Falmouth, Florence, Ft. Thomas and Williamstown, Kentucky. The merger created a system with vast resources to serve the Greater Cincinnati area, including almost 1,200 licensed beds, more than 7,300 employees, including associates from St. Elizabeth Physicians, over 1,200 physicians with privileges (which includes over 150 affiliated primary care physicians), 1,100 volunteers, 50 primary care and specialty office locations, 3 free standing imaging centers, 2 ambulatory surgery centers and 1 freestanding hospice center. The health system is sponsored by the Diocese of Covington. In 2009, the system provided more than $100 million towards Community Benefit Programs and Uncompensated Care.

Service Area

The primary service area is Boone, Campbell, Grant, Kenton and Pendleton Counties

- 2010 Estimated Population is 394,784, which is 9% of the total population of Kentucky.

- Boone County is the fastest growing county in the Commonwealth.

The secondary service area includes Bracken, Carroll, Dearborn, Gallatin, Hamilton, Harrison, Mason, Owen, and Robertson Counties.

- 2010 Estimated Population is 140,207

Lives Touched in 2010
(totals approximate)

- Almost 50,000 Inpatient Discharges
- Almost 7,800 Medicaid Inpatient Discharges
- Over 4,500 Live Births
- Over 730,000 Outpatient Visits
- Over 10,200 Inpatient Surgeries
- Over 19,200 Outpatient Surgeries
- Almost 1,000 Skilled Nursing Discharges
- Over 200,000 Emergency Department Treated and Released Visits
- Almost 25,000 Emergency Department Visits who became Inpatient Admissions or Observations